MICROBES AND DISEASES
THAT THREATEN
HUMANITY

KILLER GERMS

REVISED AND UPDATED

Barry E. Zimmerman | David J. Zimmerman

Contemporary Books

Chicago   New York   San Francisco   Lisbon   London   Madrid   Mexico City
Milan   New Delhi   San Juan   Seoul   Singapore   Sydney   Toronto

The *McGraw-Hill* Companies

Library of Congress Cataloging-in-Publication Data

Zimmerman, Barry E.
    Killer germs : microbes and diseases that threaten humanity / Barry E. Zimmerman and David J.
Zimmerman—Rev. ed.
        p.   cm.
    Includes index.
    ISBN 0-07-140926-2
    1. Communicable diseases. 2. Medical microbiology. I. Zimmerman, David J.   II. Title.

RA643.Z55   2003
616.9—dc21   2002073680

Cover photograph copyright © Todd Davidson/Getty Images

1 2 3 4 5 6 7 8 9 0   AGM/AGM   1 0 9 8 7 6 5 4 3 2

ISBN 0-07-140926-2

McGraw-Hill books are available at special quantity discounts to use as premiums and sales
promotions, or for use in corporate training programs. For more information, please write to the
Director of Special Sales, Professional Publishing, McGraw-Hill, Two Penn Plaza, New York, NY
10121-2298. Or contact your local bookstore.

This book is printed on acid-free paper.

To Marilyn and Sondra, our wives and best friends—
who are the wind beneath our wings

To Amy, Tara, and Corie, our lovely daughters—
for just being there

Thou shalt not be afraid for the terror by night,
nor for the arrow that flieth by day,
nor for the pestilence that walketh in darkness . . .

PSALM 91

Contents

Acknowledgments

MANY THANKS TO Margaret Colvin, Carol Courtney, Ann Halitsky, Bonnie Savitz, Raymond Hernandez of the Lyme Care Center, Dr. Vincent Fischetti, head of the Laboratory of Bacterial Pathogenesis and Immunology at The Rockefeller University, and Dr. David M. Klaus, Associate Director of BioServe Space Technologies, for their guidance and technical assistance.

Introduction

The beginning of health is to know the disease.

—Cervantes

THERE IS EVIDENCE of infectious disease in the fossil of a bird dating back ninety million years. A dental abscess has been found in a human ancestor between one and two million years old. (Human ancestry dates back three to five million years.) Tuberculosis was rather common six thousand years ago, during the New Stone Age, in northern Africa and Europe. Devastating plagues date back several thousand years. A smallpox plague in Rome nearly two thousand years ago killed millions of Roman citizens during a fifteen-year reign of terror. Those who survived the pestilence were often left blind or horribly disfigured. The preserved body of a Chinese noblewoman who died twenty-one hundred years ago showed scars of tuberculosis and three different kinds of worms. The conquest of the New World that began with Columbus's historic voyage was more the result of disease—smallpox along with measles and influenza—than of swords and bullets. Napoléon owed his defeat in Europe to General Typhus—which, thanks to the bite of a louse, decimated his armies—more than to any military leader. Typhus also killed three million people during World War I.

Bubonic plague—the Black Death—caused the collapse of the eastern Roman Empire in the seventh century. It killed twenty-four million Europeans in six years in the middle fourteenth century—one-third of the European population. According to Frederick Cartwright in *Disease and History*, "Mortality was so great that the Pope consecrated the river Rhône at Avignon, so that corpses flung into the river might be considered to have received Christian burial." The swine flu took the lives of at least twenty million people in six months during the winter of 1918–19. In comparison, World War I killed fifteen million people in four years.

Infectious diseases have always been with us and have shaped human history perhaps more than any other single factor. Yet they are caused by a power unseen. To quote science writer Bernard Dixon, in *Power Unseen*, "A small bacterium weighs as little as 0.000000000001 [one-trillionth] gram. A blue whale weighs about 100,000,000 [one hundred million] grams. Yet a bacterium can kill a whale." The agent of botulism food poisoning is too small to be seen with the naked eye, yet a twelve-ounce glass of the toxin it produces would kill every human being—all 6.2 billion— living on the face of the earth. As small as germs are, they rule the world.

Disease-causing organisms are a diverse group that fit into five separate categories. From simplest to most complex, they are viruses, bacteria, protozoa, fungi, and worms (see Table 1). Unlike the first four, worms are not very small; they are multicellular and, in the case of tapeworms, can be nearly as long as a tennis court.

Table 1 Human Pathogens and Parasites

Causative Agent	Diseases Caused
virus	AIDS, chicken pox, common cold, dengue fever, Ebola, flu, hantavirus, hepatitis, Lassa fever, Marburg, measles, meningitis, mononucleosis, mumps, pneumonia, rabies, rubella, West Nile, yellow fever
bacterium	bubonic plague, cholera, diphtheria, Legionnaires' disease, Lyme disease, meningitis, pneumonia, strep infections (scarlet fever, rheumatic fever, invasive strep), staph infections, tuberculosis, typhoid fever, typhus
protozoan	African sleeping sickness (trypanosomiasis), amoebic dysentery, malaria
fungus	athlete's foot, candidiasis (thrush), ringworm
worm	anisakiasis, elephantiasis, guinea worm, hookworm, river blindness, schistosomiasis, tapeworm, trichinosis

Of the five categories, those that have posed the greatest threat to developed nations and continue to do so are the viruses and bacteria—the "germ" diseases. They have been the cause of the world's great plagues and pandemics. The protozoan and worm diseases are a particular problem in developing nations, especially those with warmer climates—although viral and bacterial diseases abound there as well. All disease abounds where there is poverty, overpopulation, and inadequate sanitation and health care.

Killer Germs is a study of infectious diseases and the agents that cause them. It is divided into eleven chapters, covering several broad areas. Chapters 1 through 3 explore the history of disease, starting with the birth of germs and following the development of human thought directed at preventing and curing disease, from witchcraft to the wonder drugs. Chapters 4 and 5 focus on bacterial diseases. An entire chapter is devoted to tuberculosis, the greatest infectious-disease killer of all time. Chapters 6 through 8 investigate the viruses; they address the newly emerging, incredibly lethal hemorrhagic diseases as well as established ones such as the flu, which killed more people in six months than any other disease in human history. Chapter 9 is devoted to parasitic diseases—the protozoa and worms, which have traditionally ravaged developing nations and continue to do so. Chapter 10 is on AIDS, a viral nightmare that ravages all nations and threatens the very existence of our species. Chapter 11 is about bioterrorism, perhaps the greatest nightmare of all, because the danger is not so much a bacterium or virus but the human spirit and its ultimate capacity for evil—man's inhumanity to man.

Above all, *Killer Germs* is a book of discovery. It displays the best and worst of the human spirit. It is the story of medicine—from superstition to science at the cutting edge.

The Origin of Disease

Disease generally begins that equality which death completes.

—SAMUEL JOHNSON

DISEASE DATES BACK nearly as far as life itself. To understand its origin, we must first understand the origin of life. Our planet formed from a contracting cloud of dust and gases about four and a half billion years ago. It was a hostile world of poisonous gases, erupting volcanoes, lightning bolts, and searing radiation from a newly formed star ninety-three million miles (150 million kilometers) away. The rock that formed its crust was molten and bubbling. To quote Lynn Margulis and Dorion Sagan from *Microcosmos*:

> *During these first years . . . there was no solid ground, no oceans or lakes. . . . The planet was a molten lava fireball, burning with heat from the decay of radioactive elements in its core. The water of the Earth, shooting in steam geysers from the planet's interior, was so hot that it never fell to the surface as rain but remained high in the atmosphere, an uncondensable vapor. The atmosphere*

was thick with poisonous cyanide and formaldehyde. There was
no breathable oxygen, nor any organisms capable of breathing it.

During these first years there were no living things, period. Yet one billion years later Earth was teeming with a simple form of microbial life. Evidence of these organisms has been found in Australia and Africa in banded domes of sedimentary rock called stromatolites. These stromatolites are thought to be the fossilized remains of layered mats of bacteria that were among the earliest living things. Sediments in Greenland date back 3.85 billion years. How did bacteria form from a bubbling cauldron of lava that was the infant Earth?

Extraterrestrial Origins

There are two possibilities: (1) Life arose from nonliving matter on Earth after it cooled and became a more hospitable place (terrestrial origin), or (2) life predates Earth, and the planet was "seeded" with spores from some dark and distant corner of our galaxy (extraterrestrial origin).

The consensus among scientists distinctly favors a terrestrial origin. Most astronomers consider the conditions in deep space too hostile for life to survive—even the highly durable spore stages of certain microorganisms. In space there is no air or air pressure, and the temperature is near absolute zero (−460°F or −273°C). When approaching a habitable and seedable planet such as Earth, radiation becomes intense from the nearby sun that provides the planet with needed warmth. Without a protective atmosphere the radiation is quickly lethal to living things. In fact in 1966 the hardiest of bacteria were carried aboard the spacecraft *Gemini IX* into Earth's orbit. None survived even six hours of direct exposure to the searing ultraviolet radiation of interplanetary space.

Also, no space seeds have ever been detected in the nearly half a century we have been trekking through the cosmos. Nor have they been found as part of any meteorite or on the surface of the moon or Mars—two places where we've landed and performed tests for biological activity. If they were common enough to seed our planet within the first billion years of its creation, they should be common enough to be detected somewhere out there now. The fact that they haven't leads scientists to believe that life—and germs—originated on Earth.

Spontaneous Generation

Three hundred fifty years ago it would not have been considered wrong to believe that maggots—slithering, sluglike creatures—formed spontaneously from rotting meat; or that frogs and snakes arose spontaneously from mud at the bottom of a pond; or that dirty old rags transformed into mice and rats; or that sperm injected into cucumbers turned into people. As late as the mid-1800s people believed that microorganisms arose spontaneously from broth or gravy or other spoiling foods. The concept that life can arise from nonlife by some wondrous and inexplicable metamorphosis is known as *spontaneous generation.*

Spontaneous generation explains the origin of life on Earth easily enough. Or rather, it *accounts for* the origin of life. There is not much explanation to spontaneous generation. Nonetheless, if organisms arose spontaneously, so be it; leave the explanations to philosophers and lawyers.

Except that under controlled scientific conditions that theory did not hold up. In 1668, in a classic set of experiments, Italian physician Francesco Redi proved conclusively that maggots did not arise spontaneously from rotting meat but from the invisibly small eggs laid by meat flies on the meat. The maggots were an intermediate, caterpillarlike stage in the life cycle of the flies.

Two hundred years later the great French microbiologist Louis Pasteur would prove conclusively that microorganisms did not arise spontaneously from gravy or other spoiling foods. His experiments would sound the death knell of spontaneous generation for all time. Living things must come from other living things. Even the simplest single-celled organisms need parents—or at least a parent.

This, however, creates a catch-22. If all living things must come from living things, and there were not living things on Earth in the beginning, where did the *first* living things come from? Obviously, they could not have had parents.

Just as obviously, they must have come from nonliving stuff—but not in the sense implied by spontaneous generation. There is a vast difference in concept. Spontaneous generation has been likened to the assembly of a Boeing 707 by a hurricane in a junkyard. The creation of life was a gradual process, taking many millions of years, requiring a constant supply of high energy that is no longer available and an atmospheric composition that no longer exists. Though it probably was a global affair, occurring over different portions of the primordial Earth in shallow tidal pools, or moist sections of clay, or hot-water deep-sea vents, it was not something that happened easily. And in all likelihood it has not offered an encore performance within the last few billion years.

Evolution of Life

The tedious process of matter's increasing in complexity from inorganic to organic to living is called *chemical* or *prebiotic evolution*—evolution before life. It is not a terribly recent concept. In the 1920s A. I. Oparin in Russia and J. B. S. Haldane in England independently postulated the chemosynthesis hypothesis—that conditions on the primitive Earth favored chemical reactions that would lead to the formation of more complex molecules and ultimately to the creation of life. These conditions included a poisonous mix of gases that did not contain oxygen and abundant energy in the form of solar radiation—ultraviolet in particular—lightning discharges, and heat from Earth's gravitational contraction and the decay of radioactive elements. These high-energy conditions no longer exist and haven't for several billion years.

To test the chemosynthesis hypothesis, scientists performed experiments during the 1950s and '60s in which they re-created conditions that existed on the primitive Earth. They duplicated the primordial atmosphere and charged it with energy in the form of heat and electricity for weeks at a time. They got more than one hundred organic compounds, including amino acids and proteins, sugars, and small bits of genetic material called nucleic acids—the building blocks of life!

The success of these experiments lent strong support to the hypothesis of chemical evolution. It is likely that, in its early history, Earth's lakes and oceans became a rich organic soup. Water is an ideal medium for molecules to splash around in and react. At some point in the process certain molecules developed the ability to line up amino acids and build proteins to order, and to make copies of themselves, so that the protein-making ability could be passed on. At another point this congregation of supermolecules separated themselves into microdroplets, bound in some way by a membrane, with the internal machinery to take in and use energy and to reproduce. Life on Earth had begun.

And the living things were bacteria—the most primitive of all cells. For the next two billion years bacteria would be the sole inhabitants of Earth, a reign unparalleled by any other living thing. They have persisted twenty-five times longer than the dinosaurs and two thousand times longer than humans. There are more bacteria in a handful of soil or inside your mouth than the total number of people that have ever lived. A single sneeze can carry with it a million bacteria. They make up 90 percent of the weight of human feces. Your body contains more bacterial cells than human cells—one hundred times as many! And they are found everywhere on earth—in the deepest oceans, on the highest mountain tops, even wafting along on high-altitude clouds.

The earliest cells were not initially parasitic. They lived free, feasting on the wealth of food in the seas, compliments of chemosynthesis. But they mutated in insidious ways and soon learned to invade free-living cells and cause disease—and changed forever the way life went on. Those that did not become parasitic evolved, in time, into all other living things—even the viruses, which are much simpler than the simplest bacteria. (Bacteria are the simplest cells, but viruses are not cells; they are merely a collection of molecules.) According to Rita Coswell of the University of Maryland, there are between three hundred thousand and one million different species of bacteria. Most are not pathogenic. But the handful that are, along with the viruses and parasites that they spawned, have caused untold misery and have dictated the course of human events.

2

Germs and Disease: A Brief History

There are some remedies worse than the disease.

—Publilius Syrus

Languor seizes the body from bad ventilation.

—Ovid

Witchcraft, Retribution, and the Humor of It All

In 1831 a mad wolf charged through a small village in eastern France, jaws snapping, fangs bared, a poisonous lather spilling from its jowls. The wolf had just attacked the village blacksmith, badly mangling him. The man would survive the wounds; they would heal. In several months, however, he would be dead of rabies.

A boy of nine went home that day and asked his father, "What makes a wolf or a dog mad? Why do people die when mad dogs bite them?" His father, a village tanner, replied, "Perhaps a devil got into the wolf. If God wills you are to die, you will die." The boy who asked the questions was

Louis Pasteur, and over the next half century he would answer them and many others.

Ignorance of the cause of disease prevailed throughout most of human history. People became ill because evil spirits entered their bodies. Through incantation and ritual dances and the use of various potions and arcane procedures, medicine men and witch doctors sought to drive out these spirits. If a patient whose body had been smeared with animal feces recovered, the shaman was revered as a great healer. If the patient died, it was not the fault of the doctor; the patient was paying for the sins that he had committed. King Tutankhamen, who died prematurely of tuberculosis, his lungs eaten away by the disease, was presumably paying for the sins of his father. It was a primitive concept of disease as divine retribution. People lived, they suffered, and they died. Humanity was virtually helpless in the face of the great plagues that periodically swept the land, killing or disabling millions of people.

Despite all of this futility, human ingenuity was never at a loss for preventive and curative measures. In Russia, to ward off pestilence, the townsfolk would hitch four widows to a plowshare and cut a furrow around their village in the dead of night (three widows would never do). King Louis XIV of France endured more than two thousand enemas during his seventy-two-year reign, to combat disease and to promote good health. (Known as *le Roi Soleil*—the Sun King—he might well have been called the "Moon" King, or Public Enema Number One.) George Washington, suffering from a sore throat and respiratory infection, was the recipient of "state-of-the-art" medical treatment in 1799. He was given a poisonous compound of mercury, by both mouth and injection. He was forced to ingest a poisonous white salt that made him perspire and vomit. Caustic poultices were applied to his body that made his skin blister. He was forced to inhale vinegar vapors that burned his lungs and raised blisters in his throat, to counteract the blisters of infection. As a final affront, more than five pints (2.4 liters) of blood were drained from his body. (An average-size male has ten or eleven pints—the volume of oil in the crankcase of your car.) All to no avail. He died shortly afterward—perhaps as much from the cure as from the illness.

The practice of removing blood from the body to combat disease was particularly popular. It was called *bloodletting* and was performed well into the nineteenth century. The treatment was based on a theory dating back to the teachings of Hippocrates in the fifth century B.C. People believed that the human body contained four fluids, or humors: blood, phlegm, yellow bile, and black bile. Hippocrates considered disease to be the result of an imbalance among these fluids. Sometimes the body could successfully restore the balance by itself, as evidenced by natural recovery from disease. At other times, however, the body needed help from a physician. Drawing blood from a patient was a favored approach (which was usually accomplished by cutting into a vein or applying leeches). In replenishing the lost blood, the body would somehow be stimulated to restore the proper balance of body fluids.

Before Washington, King Louis XV of France was the unfortunate recipient of similar medical wisdom. On the morning of April 27, 1774, he awoke quite ill. His body ached, and he was dizzy and feverish. Within a week ugly, pus-filled sores erupted on his face and neck and soon spread to the rest of his body. They filled his mouth and throat and caused great pain. He was suffering from a disease called smallpox, the terror of Europe and the New World. The royal medical team gathered and decided there was only one thing to do: the French monarch must be bled. He was exsanguinated until he lost consciousness (which was standard operating procedure); four large basinfuls of blood were removed from his body. No one can say whether the action hastened or delayed his death, which occurred on May 10. Such was the state of affairs in the medical community little more than two hundred years ago.

There were exceptions to this school of ignorance, but the perceptions of those with more progressive beliefs did not lead quickly to change. The germ theory was not formed all at once, like Athena springing full-grown and in full armor from the head of Zeus. To quote René Dubos, the great microbiologist and discoverer of the first antibiotic to be produced commercially: "The belief that microbes can cause disease had emerged as an abstract concept—a hunch—long before it was possible to state the facts clearly or to test them by experiment. Over many years, the theory evolved progressively from a vague awareness to the level of precise understanding" (*Pasteur and Modern Science*).

The roots of this understanding date back thousands of years. Virgil and Varro, citizens of the Roman Empire, said that some diseases were caused by invisible seeds. These seeds flew about in the air and were breathed in through the nose and mouth, causing infection and death. Sixteen hundred years later an Italian physician, Girolamo Fracastoro, suggested that syphilis was transmitted sexually by a *contagium vivum*, or "living agent." He outlined the different modes through which these living agents, and those of other diseases as well, could be spread: direct contact with an infected person, handling of contaminated materials, and breathing in infected air. About two hundred years later, in the mid-1700s, the Austrian physician Marcus von Plenciz theorized that not only were diseases caused by invisible living organisms but that each disease had its own particular culprit.

What marvelous insight. In the face of superstition and ignorance, of evil spirits and bloodletting, these men stood out as solitary candles in the darkness. Their tragic failing was that they did not offer proof. They did not subject their hunches and theories to controlled scientific experimentation. They did not collect data to back their claims. But there were great scientists on the horizon who would, people who would establish, through rigorous analysis, the germ theory of disease and usher in the Golden Age of Bacteriology—a span of about fifty years from the mid-1800s to the turn of the century.

Seeing the Invisible

The discovery of microbes and their role in disease awaited the invention of the microscope. Without the ability to see microbes, the most elegant theories involving them were conjecture. To quote Rosalyn Yalow, a Noble Prize–winning medical researcher, "New truths become evident when new tools become available." The microscope opened a world of new truths. The human eye cannot see objects with a diameter smaller than about $1/250$ inch (100 micrometers). Most germs that cause disease are at least fifty times smaller.

It is difficult to ascribe the invention of the microscope to any one person. Magnifying lenses were ground from glass as far back as ancient Grecian and Roman times. Credit for putting lenses together to increase magnification to "microscopic" powers is generally given to two Dutch spectacle makers, Hans Janssen and his son, Zacharius, circa 1598. Seventy-five years later a simple, unassuming, poorly educated dry-goods dealer used magnifying lenses to discover the world of microbes. He was Dutch, and his name was Antonie van Leeuwenhoek.

Leeuwenhoek ground 419 individual lenses from which he constructed 247 simple microscopes (which used only one lens) that could magnify up to 270 times. He trained these microscopes on everything that caught his fancy: the bodies of many insects and bugs; the stomach contents, feces, and semen of a menagerie of animals including humans; stagnant pools of water; spoiling food; the plaque on people's teeth, and so on. He was the first person to see sperm cells (his own), blood cells, and a veritable zoo of protozoa and bacteria (but not viruses—they were too small even for his magic lenses). Some of the animalcules in his zoo did somersaults, some glided smoothly through their liquid surroundings, and some did not move at all. Some were round, while others were long and thin or corkscrew-shaped.

For fifty years, until his death at age ninety-one, Leeuwenhoek observed his world of microbes, his "wretched beasties" as he called them, reporting his findings to the Royal Society of London, an organization established for the dissemination of scientific information. The American Society for Microbiology prints a picture of Leeuwenhoek on the cover of its monthly periodical, the *Journal of Bacteriology*, and he is generally regarded as the father of microbiology.

After Leeuwenhoek died in 1723, the field of microbiology and disease—of science in general—entered a period of dormancy that lasted the better part of 150 years. There were a few notable exceptions, moments of discovery and advance. One concerned the disease that claimed the life of poor King Louis—smallpox. It was a thoroughly horrid illness that spread easily from person to person by direct or indirect contact or through the air. It killed up to 40 percent of the people who contracted it, by infiltrating and destroying their kidneys, heart, or brain. Those who survived were often left with serious kidney damage or terribly disfigured from scars and deep pits—especially on the face—that remained after the smallpox sores healed. It was also a leading cause of blindness.

Genoese explorer Christopher Columbus brought smallpox to the New World in 1492, and it has since killed hundreds of millions of people in North and South America. Hernando Cortés of Spain brought an infected slave with him when he conquered Mexico in 1520, and two years later 3.5 million naive (never before exposed) and vulnerable Aztec natives were dead of smallpox. By the eighteenth century it was killing four hundred thousand people in Europe every year. Abraham Lincoln was probably infected with smallpox when he gave the Gettysburg Address. As recently as 1950 smallpox killed more than one million people in India. In 1967 it was still infecting between ten and fifteen million people worldwide and killing more than two million. *Today's Science on File* (November 1999) cites that "From 1900 to 1980, smallpox killed 500 million people—more than all of the century's wars, the 1918 influenza epidemic and the AIDS epidemic combined. Only malaria may have caused more deaths." Yet a method of preventing the disease has been known for more than two hundred years.

A Milkmaid's Tale

A procedure called *variolation* (from the Latin for smallpox, *variola*), or inoculation, had been practiced for many hundreds of years. It developed from the knowledge that people who got smallpox and recovered from it never got it again. They became immune. Doctors reasoned that if they could intentionally infect their patients with a mild form of the disease, they could, in turn, make them immune. It was called "sowing" or "buying" the pox.

As early as the eleventh century, Chinese doctors sowed the pox by making a powder from the dried scabs of victims with mild cases of smallpox and then having their healthy patients inhale the powder through straws. In other societies doctors made small incisions in the flesh of their patients and rubbed the scab powder directly into the wound. This method of inoculation—called *ingrafting*—became popular in Europe and Great Britain in the seventeenth and eighteenth centuries and was practiced by peasantry and royalty alike. In fact the family of Louis XV had themselves inoculated shortly after the death of the king. Across the Atlantic, among the British colonies in America, inoculation was also quite popular.

But the procedure was not without serious risk. A weak-acting germ in one individual is not necessarily weak-acting in another. Nearly as often as not, the inoculation caused a disfiguring, blinding, or fatal case of the disease rather than the mild one that was anticipated. Though the risk did not discourage the practice, inoculation was clearly not the answer to smallpox prevention.

The breakthrough came one day as a milkmaid was being examined by an apprentice surgeon named Edward Jenner in the rural county of Gloucestershire, England. When young Jenner suggested that the woman was suffering from smallpox, she replied confidently, "I cannot take the smallpox, for I have had the cowpox."

Gloucestershire was dairy land, and a disease called cowpox periodically afflicted the cattle that grazed in the pastures. (Two other similar diseases were swinepox and horsepox.) It caused sores on the udders of the dairy cows and spread easily by contact to the maids who milked them. In humans it was a discomforting ailment, causing fever, nausea, and painful sores on the hands and wrists. It was not, however, a serious illness. It did not blind, disfigure, or kill. But it did confer immunity to smallpox. If one had "had the cowpox" one could not "take the smallpox."

While other doctors considered it an old wives' tale, Jenner saw the link between cowpox infection and smallpox prevention. In 1789 he inoculated his ten-month-old son, Edward Jr., with the pus from a swinepox sore. A while later he inoculated the boy with smallpox matter. The child did not take ill with smallpox—he had developed immunity. But Jenner did not publicize the achievement, and its significance was not appreciated in the medical community.* Seven years later, however, Jenner would perform an experiment that would lend him immortality, save countless millions of lives, and eradicate a disease for the first and only time in the history of mankind.

On that day Jenner removed matter from the cowpox sore of a dairy-maid named Sarah Nelmes and scratched it into the skin on the arm of an eight-year-old boy, James Phipps. Seven weeks later Jenner inoculated the young lad with smallpox matter. Nothing happened. He inoculated Phipps with deadly smallpox matter more than twenty times over the next twenty-five years, and every time . . . nothing happened.

The procedure of injecting cowpox matter into a person to induce immunity to smallpox was coined *vaccination*, after *vacca*, the Latin term for "cow." The injection itself was called a *vaccine*.

---

*Interestingly, Edward Jenner Jr. would become a sickly child with mild mental retardation and would die at age twenty-one of tuberculosis. It has been speculated that secondary infection from the smallpox vaccine may have caused these problems.

The response to vaccination was immediate and widespread. By 1800 several hundred thousand people had been vaccinated. Compulsory vaccination laws were established. In 1801 smallpox vaccine was sent to President Thomas Jefferson, who had himself and his family vaccinated, as well as some neighbors and Indians. According to Peter Radetsky, author of *The Invisible Invaders*, when Jenner died in 1823 he was the most honored man of his time; a cottage he built for young Mr. Phipps—whom he looked after for twenty-seven years until his own death—is now the Jenner Museum. He had introduced to the world the medical procedure of immunization. One hundred eighty-one years after his historic vaccination of James Phipps, in October 1977 in Somalia, the last naturally occurring case of smallpox would be reported—the result of an intensive ten-year, $300 million immunization program implemented by the World Health Organization (WHO). After three thousand or more years of infecting humanity, the world would no longer take the smallpox, for it had been given Jenner's cowpox. (Unlike for most other diseases, humans are the only natural reservoir for the smallpox virus. This is important; it lends the disease to eradication.)

The smallpox virus happens to be very stable in nature. Though the disease has been eradicated, and the vaccine is no longer a part of immunization protocol, there are scientists who feel archaeologists should still be immunized. Because of the stability of the virus, mummies or other preserved bodies thousands of years old might contain smallpox virus or genetic fragments that are viable and infectious.

There is an interesting subscript to the smallpox saga. Although the disease has been wiped out, the germ that causes it has not. All samples of the virus have been transferred to two sites—the U.S. Centers for Disease Control and Prevention (CDC) in Atlanta, Georgia, and the State Research Center of Virology and Biotechnology (called Vector) in Kotsovo, Russia— where they remain in a frozen state. Fierce debate is being waged concerning the fate of these remaining stocks. Some feel that the virus must be destroyed lest people become infected accidentally or through the action of terrorist groups or nations at war. Others argue that much can be learned from studying the virus. It may help scientists understand the nature of viral infection and provide methods to combat other diseases. There is even talk of using the stuff of the smallpox vaccine as a vehicle for an AIDS vaccine: genetic material from a disabled AIDS virus would be placed into the stable and safe vaccinia (cowpox) virus. In the meantime, geneticists have made copies of parts of the smallpox virus, which they say are not in themselves pathogenic but may store useful information about smallpox infection. They have also mapped the entire genome of three strains of the virus so that if the remaining stocks are ultimately destroyed the genetic information they contain will be safeguarded.

The virus has endured several stays of execution to this point. In 1986 a committee of WHO experts unanimously recommended destroying the virus, setting December 30, 1993, as the date; it was subsequently postponed to June 30, 1995. That date passed without final resolution. In January 24, 1996, the governing board of WHO recommended destruction by June 30, 1999. In 1998, seventy-four of seventy-nine countries responding to a WHO survey wanted the virus destroyed, which included the United States but not Russia. Subsequently, after a study by the Clinton administration into the consequences of making variola (smallpox) extinct, the United States has changed its position, and now favors additional research. A major reason is the fear that rogue nations with ties to terrorist groups may have secretly secured stockpiles of the virus, and plan to use it against the United States and its allies. To be without a living specimen to study and use for vaccine preparation would put us at a distinct disadvantage. (See Chapter 11, "Bioterrorism," for a full account of smallpox as a weapon of bioterror.)

With neither country officially storing the virus now wanting to destroy it, WHO has again delayed its destruction to the end of 2002. If that ultimately happens, it will be the first time in history that a living thing will purposefully and with full knowledge of the consequences be made extinct. The method of extinction will be to heat the virus to death in a pressure cooker at 248°F (120°C) for forty-five minutes. The dead germs will then be incinerated.

The year before Jenner died, a man was born who would usher in a new age of discovery in medicine and disease. He was an impudent and argumentative fellow with a scornful cockiness. He was an impetuous experimenter and at times jumped to conclusions that were ill-advised. But he was brilliant. He was Louis Pasteur, the nine-year-old boy who had asked his father why people die when mad dogs bite them. Part of his story is an extension of the work of Jenner and immunization.

Chance Favors the Prepared Mind

The year was 1880, and Pasteur was fifty-eight years old. He was already famous for having saved the wine and silk industries of France (by demonstrating that microbes spoiled wine and killed silkworms) and for establishing a causal link between microbes and infectious disease. He hobbled noticeably from paralysis of his left side, due to a stroke suffered several years earlier. Yet his greatest accomplishments lay ahead.

At the time, Pasteur happened to be working with a microbe that killed chickens and other birds by infecting them with a disease called chicken cholera. (This is not the same cholera that afflicts humans and that has been responsible for devastating plagues in India and other countries with poor public health and sanitation.) He would culture the germs in a chicken broth and then feed them to unsuspecting chickens on bits of bread or inject them. Invariably within several days the chickens were dead. Pasteur's laboratory benches became cluttered with abandoned cultures of chicken cholera. One day, instead of throwing away these old tubes of chicken soup, which was his practice, he decided to inject them into a batch of healthy chickens. To his surprise the chickens did not die. They got sick, their feathers ruffled, their appetites flagged, but they recovered. Pasteur did not take particular notice. It was known that in nature animals sometimes recovered from typically fatal diseases. Why not in the laboratory as well?

Without further thought about it, Pasteur closed up the laboratory and went on summer vacation with his family. Weeks later he was back at work, feeding his chickens a deadly brew of chicken soup.

"Bring up some new birds and get them ready," he told his laboratory assistant.

"But we have only a couple of unused chickens left, Mr. Pasteur," the assistant replied. "Remember, you used the last ones before you went away—you injected the old cultures into them, and they got sick but didn't die."

For want of a fresh batch, Pasteur decided to inject these "used" birds. He inoculated them with a particularly virulent strain of chicken cholera bacteria. They did not die. To his astonishment, they did not even get ill. The few new chickens that he had injected died within a day or two. It was indeed puzzling.

Then, in what must have been a blinding flash of insight, Pasteur realized what had happened. The germs that he had inoculated into the chickens before he went on vacation had become weaker upon standing. They
could no longer kill. But they *could* confer immunity. Pasteur had created
the world's second vaccine. It was the first vaccine made from the germ
that caused the disease rather than from a different but closely related germ.
Pasteur's vaccine had the distinct advantage of universality. No other disease was like smallpox, which had a ready-made weaker cousin in the cowpox germ. But all germs—or certainly many—could be weakened, or
attenuated, by one method or another to provide a vaccine.

Pasteur's discovery of the chicken cholera vaccine was fortuitous, but
chance favors the prepared mind (a theme that will repeat itself). To turn
accident into discovery, to see the link between chickens that would not
die and a broad method of immunizing against disease, took genius. And
Pasteur was just warming up.

A Sheepish Situation

It was now 1881. Pasteur had turned his discerning eye from chicken
cholera to a dreadful disease called anthrax. It was caused by a rod-shaped
bacterium (called a bacillus) and killed sheep, other farm animals, and
humans. Painstakingly Pasteur worked in his laboratory, weakening the
anthrax bacilli in stages so that some killed mice but not guinea pigs, others killed guinea pigs but not rabbits, and still others killed rabbits but not
sheep. By injecting appropriately weakened microbes into sheep and cattle, he conferred upon them immunity to the disease. He reported his successes to the Academy of Sciences in Paris.

The members were not entirely impressed. More than a few doubted
Pasteur's claims. He was, in fact, challenged to perform a public experiment in which he would demonstrate the effectiveness of his anthrax vaccine. The event was greatly publicized and became something of a media
circus. It was the first public trial of an experimental vaccine. A flock of
newspaper reporters were in attendance, as well as a host of VIPs from the
scientific community. The experiment began on May 5, 1881, on a farm
called Pouilly-le-Fort. Twenty-four sheep, one goat, and six cows were vaccinated with a weakened culture of anthrax bacillus. On May 17 they were
injected with a somewhat stronger dose. On May 31 they were injected

with a full-strength, highly virulent strain of the germ. Twenty-four sheep, one goat, and four cows that had not been vaccinated were injected as well. After two days the unvaccinated sheep and goat were all dead and the four cows were dying; the vaccinated animals were all healthy. Pasteur had met the challenge. Vaccination of farm animals against anthrax soon became a widely established practice. In 2001, vaccination was offered to those at risk after a bioterror incident in which anthrax spores were found at several U.S. mail distribution centers and on Capitol Hill.

Mad Dogs and Frenchmen

Despite his triumphs over chicken cholera and anthrax, Pasteur's antirabies treatment is generally regarded as his greatest triumph. Unlike the chicken cholera and anthrax vaccines, which were designed to save the lives of birds, sheep, and horses (though anthrax did infect and kill humans as well), the rabies vaccine was designed to save the lives of people. Unlike nearly every other disease, mortality from rabies was 100 percent and it was a positively awful way to die. Radetsky, in *The Invisible Invaders*, describes the progress of the disease:

> *First comes fever, then depression, then restlessness that turns into uncontrollable excitement. The muscles of the throat convulse, and saliva froths and runs down the chin, causing great thirst. But even the smallest sip of water may produce convulsions and more thirst. In the later stages of the disease, the mere sight of water can bring on convulsions and paralysis—thus the archaic name for the disease,* hydrophobia, *"fear of water."*

It was after his successful demonstration of anthrax immunization that Pasteur turned his attention to this dreaded disease that made dogs and wolves mad. "I have always been haunted by the cries of those victims of the mad wolf that came down the street of Arbois when I was a little boy." At the age of sixty he began sticking his hand into the frothing mouths of rabid dogs, whose jaws were held open by his dutiful assistants, to draw off small amounts of saliva with which to culture the rabies microbe.

But to Pasteur's surprise and consternation, the microbe could not be grown in an artificial medium. None of his chicken or beef broths would do. The microbe could not be seen either. Pasteur did not know it, but he was looking for a virus. Viruses cannot be cultured outside of living tissue, and they were far too small for Pasteur's microscopes.

Without the ability to culture the "bug," a continuous supply of mad animals would be necessary. After all, to make a vaccine Pasteur needed the germs. The problem was that mad dogs or wolves—or even foxes or raccoons, which were also sources of rabies—were not easy to come by. So Pasteur decided to culture the germ inside healthy animals. When a mad dog was brought to his laboratory, he would put it in a cage with healthy dogs and allow it to bite them. But it didn't always work. If four dogs were bitten, two might develop rabies, and it took months to happen. Clearly this was not acceptable.

Then one day an idea came to Pasteur. The general symptoms of the disease suggested that it affected the nervous system. If germs from the ground-up brains of an animal just dead of rabies could be injected directly into the brain of a healthy dog. . . . But the idea of such a thing was repugnant to him.

Pasteur's assistant Pierre-Paul-Émile Roux (who would go on to do important work with the childhood killer diphtheria), was not so squeamish. Without telling Pasteur, he proceeded to drill a hole in the skull of a dog and inoculate the deadly rabies virus directly into its brain (a process called *trephination*). If done properly, trephination is not at all painful to the animal. Roux convinced Pasteur of this, and the problem of culturing the rabies virus was solved.

For years Pasteur cultured the germ in trephined dogs and tried various ways to weaken it for use in a vaccine. He met with success by removing a bit of spinal cord from a rabbit dead of rabies and drying it in a germ-proof bottle for fourteen days. This made the virus harmless. Pasteur developed a protocol for rabies prophylaxis in which he prepared progressively stronger cultures of the germ by drying it for one-day-shorter periods of time. The procedure involved fourteen injections over fourteen days. It worked well on all of his laboratory dogs. At the end of the vaccination period full-strength rabies virus had no effect on the animals.

Despite these successes, it is unlikely that Pasteur ever would have tested his vaccine on a healthy individual, though he received many requests. The risks were too great and the nature of the disease too horrible. Instead he proposed to vaccinate every dog in France—all 2.5 million of them. This idea quickly proved impractical.

The question of how to use his vaccine to benefit mankind remained unanswered until July 6, 1885, when a frightened woman burst into his laboratory with her nine-year-old son, Joseph Meister. The boy had been bitten viciously in more than a dozen places on his hands and legs by a rabid dog, and death from rabies was virtually certain. But the disease acted slowly. Symptoms did not usually appear until a month or more after the bite. (The incubation period in humans ranges from one week to more than a year, with thirty to fifty days being average.) Perhaps the vaccine could be used as a treatment rather than a prevention. Joseph Meister's mother pleaded with Pasteur to save her son's life. And he did. On July 7, sixty hours after little Joseph had been bitten, Pasteur gave him his first injection, increasing the strength of the vaccine over ten consecutive days and fourteen injections. The rest is history. Pasteur had performed his most dramatic feat at the age of sixty-three.

Within fifteen months after saving the life of Joseph Meister, Pasteur had vaccinated no fewer than 2,490 people, including 19 Russian peasants who had been bitten by a mad wolf and who were certain to die without his treatment. All but three of the peasants survived. The czar of Russia, in an outpouring of gratitude, sent Pasteur one hundred thousand francs to start the building of a research facility in his name—what is now the world-renowned Pasteur Institute, where, among other discoveries, scientists first reported identification of the AIDS virus. Pasteur's general methods of rabies prophylaxis are still in use today. (Currently, six injections are usually given over a three-month period. The procedure is also much less painful than it originally was.) The major sources of human infection in the United States today are wild animals—raccoons, skunks, foxes, and bats. The disease is rare in dogs, due to widespread vaccination. Cats are the most common domestic animals that contract rabies.

Although rabies is relatively rare in the United States, it is endemic in developing nations such as Asia and Africa, and kills forty thousand to seventy thousand people each year worldwide. About ten million people receive postexposure treatment annually, and pre-exposure vaccination is recommended for those who will be living in high-risk regions of the world for more than a month.

There is a rather poignant epilogue to the rabies story. In his later years Meister became gatekeeper of the Pasteur Institute in Paris, which housed the burial crypt of Louis Pasteur. In 1940, fifty-five years after his life had been spared, Nazi invaders demanded that he open Pasteur's crypt. Rather than do so, he committed suicide.

Vaccines against many diseases have been developed in the wake of Pasteur's achievements, using his methods as a model. For diphtheria and tetanus, a vaccine was developed using not the weakened microbe that causes the disease but a modified form of the harmful toxin it produces (called a *toxoid*). For other diseases the vaccine consisted of microbes that were killed rather than weakened—usually by heat or chemical treatment. Jonas Salk's 1954 polio vaccine was such an example. It immunized against a crippling viral disease that afflicted children in particular, including the young Franklin D. Roosevelt.

Many diseases for which vaccines have been developed still kill millions of people—especially in developing nations—because of the high cost, in both money and manpower, of implementing vaccination programs.

The American Academy of Pediatrics, as of 2002, recommends the following child immunization schedule—beginning preferably before the age of two years, if children are to be protected during their most vulnerable period:

- Hepatitis B—a blood-borne, viral disease that infects the liver and is associated with liver cancer [vaccine: Hep B]
- Diphtheria, tetanus (lockjaw), pertussis (whooping cough) [vaccine: DTaP]
- Polio (infantile paralysis)—a viral disease that affects the nervous system [vaccine: IPV or OVP]
- Measles, mumps, rubella (German Measles) [vaccine: MMR]
- Varicella (chicken pox)—approved in the United States in 1995 [vaccine: Varivax]
- Pneumococcus—causes a bacterial pneumonia, sinusitis, ear infections, and serious blood poisoning; approved in the United States in 2000 [vaccine: PCV or Prevnar]

- *Haemophilus influenzae* type b—causes a bacterial pneumonia that often leads to meningitis; approved in the United States in 1989 [vaccine: HiB]
- Influenza (the "flu")—for children with certain risk factors, such as asthma, sickle cell disease, HIV, diabetes

Many city and state departments of health require an immunization protocol that includes all or most of these diseases before a child may enter public or private school.

There has been some controversy regarding vaccination, especially of children. Various public-interest groups have campaigned against its widespread use. Citizens for Healthcare Freedom cites, for instance, that the chance of a serious adverse reaction to the DTaP vaccine is one in 1,750, while the chance of dying from pertussis each year is one in several million. They also note (according to several National Vaccine Information Center investigations) that serious adverse reactions to vaccination are drastically underreported, and that such reactions may be a major contributing factor to the sudden infant death syndrome (SIDS).

As a counterpoint, the American Council on Science and Health (ACSH) released two publications in November 2001 that present strong evidence that vaccinations are safe as well as effective and urge Americans to continue immunizing their children according to national health guidelines. Says Dr. Gilbert L. Ross, medical director of ACSH: "The benefits of childhood vaccination are more evident today than at any time in the past fifty years." As an example, during the 1980s *Haemophilus influenzae* type B was the leading cause of meningitis in American infants. Then the HiB vaccine came out, and HiB meningitis virtually disappeared. Vaccination has been and remains the most effective public health intervention for protecting children from illness and death by infectious disease.

In New York City, Mayor Rudolph Giuliani declared May 1995 Immunization Month in an effort to get all parents to immunize their children. More than half a dozen years later, up to 70 percent of children in some urban areas are still inadequately immunized.

To simplify vaccination, combination vaccines are being developed. HiB is already being included in the MMR vaccine, and a combination hepatitis A, B, and C vaccine is in the works. There is, however, a growing childhood vaccine shortage due to pharmaceutical companies bailing out of vaccine production because of lawsuits resulting from adverse patient reactions to vaccination and because making vaccines is simply not especially profitable.

Doctors of Death

It is difficult to assess the contribution of Pasteur to microbiology, to medicine, and to humanity.* Before his work on immunization he was busy demonstrating the link between germs and disease. He showed that silkworms die because germs get inside them and multiply. He could not help noticing that whenever a sheep or cow died of anthrax, or a bird of chicken cholera, there were curious microbes multiplying in their bloodstreams—but never in the blood of healthy animals. He intimated that infectious diseases in humans must also be caused by these "malignant microbes." During the Franco-Prussian War (1870–71), Pasteur convinced doctors to boil their instruments before using them on wounded soldiers and to steam their bandages. This practice greatly reduced the presence of microbes and the incidence of death by infection from battle injuries and wound surgery. (These infections were caused by several types of bacteria, among them staphylococcus, which also caused boils and abscesses; streptococcus, which also caused sore throats; and clostridium, which turned the wound gangrenous.)

Germ-Free Surgery

In Europe the professors and students of the medical colleges were beginning to get excited and to quarrel over Pasteur's ideas on germs and disease. News of Pasteur's theories reached England, where a Scottish surgeon, Joseph Lister, was practicing his craft. Surgery had recently entered a new era with the development of anesthesia. In 1846 an American dentist, William Thomas Green Morton, performed facial surgery to remove a tumor from a patient who was inhaling a mixture of air and ether. The patient felt no pain during the operation. This was a remarkable

---

*Doubt has been cast in recent years regarding the originality of Pasteur's research. A study of his laboratory notebooks by some historians of science has shown a discrepancy between his research data and his published results.

accomplishment, allowing doctors to do many surgical procedures that before could not be done because of the resulting shock induced by pain.

Unfortunately, the patient often died days or weeks later from infection, known as *surgical sepsis*. As surgery in the operating room increased, so did death in the recovery room. Anesthesia, in fact, was prevented from having its deserved impact on medical practice because of this. The threat of infection made it impossible to operate within the body cavity, except under the direst circumstances—a burst appendix, a ruptured spleen. In many hospitals eight out of ten surgical patients died from subsequent infection. Sir Frederick Treves, a respected English doctor and writer of the late 1800s, summed up the attitude of the public toward hospitals and healing in the following, from his essay "The Old Receiving Room":

> *I was instructed by my surgeon to obtain a woman's permission for an operation on her daughter. The operation was one of no great magnitude. I discussed the procedure with the mother in great detail and, I trust, in a sympathetic and hopeful manner. After I had finished my discourse I asked her if she would consent to the performance of the operation. She replied: "Oh! it is all very well to talk about consenting, but who is to pay for the funeral?"*

Sir James Simpson, the Scottish obstetrician who introduced chloroform anesthesia, said correctly in 1867, in an article titled "Hospitalism," "The man laid on the operating table . . . is exposed to more chances of death than the English soldier on the field of Waterloo." The surgeon came to expect the sight of pus and inflammation and the nauseating stench of putrefying flesh in the postsurgical wards.

That people died routinely of wound infection bothered Lister very much. He had read of the work of Pasteur and under his influence proposed that microbes were the cause of postsurgical infection. To reduce the presence of these microbes, Lister used a solution of carbolic acid (called *phenol*) that was known to have bactericidal effects. It was used, in fact, for the treatment of sewage and human waste. Lister sprayed the air in the operating theaters with a fine mist of phenol. He soaked surgical instruments in it and had surgeons wash their hands with it. Death from surgical sepsis declined dramatically. Lister had introduced antiseptic surgery. In his honor we use Listerine antiseptic mouthwash and call certain rod-shaped and occasionally pathogenic bacteria *Listeria*. Today antiseptic agents more effective than phenol are used in hospitals, and doctors and nurses wear gloves, masks, and gowns and "scrub" thoroughly before any surgical procedure.

Though sepsis deaths greatly diminished with antiseptic ("against germs") and aseptic ("no germs") procedures and with the advent of antibiotics, sepsis in hospital wards, especially intensive care units—where patients have nonfunctional or minimally functional immune systems—still presents a problem. In American hospitals alone, twenty patients an hour will die of sepsis this year. We must become increasingly vigilant of nosocomial, or hospital-contracted, infections, which afflict two million Americans annually, killing 95,000, at a cost of nearly $500 billion. It has been said that the most dangerous place for a sick person to be is in a hospital.

Death in the Delivery Room

The influence of Pasteur and his germ theory of disease had created a favorable climate for Lister's work toward antiseptic medicine. This was not the case when Ignaz Semmelweis practiced medicine in Vienna only twenty years earlier.

Semmelweis was trained in medicine at the Vienna University Medical School, where he graduated in 1844. He decided to study obstetrics and was appointed assistant to Johann Klein, professor of obstetrics at the university. In this capacity he performed autopsies on women who had died of childbed fever—an often fatal infection of the uterus that afflicted women after delivery. In some hospitals as many as one in four women who gave birth died of childbed fever, which was also known as puerperal fever. Most doctors dismissed puerperal fever as an epidemic disease caused by a specific agent of unknown origin, like smallpox. Others said it was caused by "bad air," a reactionary concept from the days of witchcraft and superstition.

Semmelweis, in the meantime, noticed something very puzzling at the Vienna General Hospital, where women were routinely delivering and dying. In those wards where obstetricians and medical students delivered the babies, an average of six hundred to eight hundred mothers died of childbed fever each year. Where midwives delivered a similar number of babies, the annual death rate was sixty—less than one-tenth! Mothers who delivered their babies at home had an even lower mortality, nearly zero.

A tragic accident provided Semmelweis with the solution to the puzzle. The head of forensic pathology at the Vienna Medical School was accidentally injured during an autopsy and died subsequently of an overwhelming wound infection. Semmelweis noticed remarkable similarities between the course of the pathologist's illness and that of childbed fever. Then he realized what was happening. Childbed fever was not caused by a mysterious epidemic or by miasmic air. It was a wound infection of the uterus caused by the contaminated hands of doctors who were performing autopsies and then delivering babies. As they left the autopsy rooms—the death houses—they carried with them the "cadaver particles" of the corpses they had handled and transferred these deadly particles to the torn and infection-susceptible wombs of postpartum women. They *smelled* of the death houses; they reeked of the putrid cadavers they had dissected. And they carried death with them into the delivery rooms. Ironically, it was a smell they had come to be proud of—the hospital odor of the time-honored physician. The dirtier and more crusted with blood a surgeon's operating coat, the greater evidence of his prowess.

Semmelweis considered childbed fever a transmissible but not contagious disease. The cadaver particles, as he called them, were not one particular type of germ but a variety of agents that could infect a wound and lead to generalized sepsis. (Staphylococcus and streptococcus, as mentioned earlier, were two common causative agents, along with half a dozen others.) Using his authority as Klein's assistant, Semmelweis ordered all obstetricians and their assistants to wash their hands thoroughly in a solution of chlorinated water until they no longer smelled of cadavers. The results were dramatic. In the months before this prophylaxis, in 1847, the death rate from childbed fever among doctor-delivered babies was 18.3 percent. One year after the prophylaxis the death rate plummeted to 1.2 percent. Apparently childbed fever would no longer pose a serious threat to women giving birth.

Astonishingly, this was not the case. Part of the blame must be placed on the medical community in Austria at the time. Although there was a brotherhood of young and progressive doctors who were politically active and championed the ideas of Semmelweis and other revolutionaries, the "elder statesmen" in the medical profession carried greater political clout. They were conservative in their views, were slow to accept change, and, most important, were loath to admit that but for the simple act of washing their hands countless women had suffered and died.

Some of the blame, however, must also be placed on Semmelweis himself. He did little to promote his beliefs. He did not publish his results on childbed fever clearly and fully. He was abrasive, arrogant, and insulting to those who would hold his destiny in their hands (quite literally). In open letters he accused the highly respected professors of obstetrics at Vienna and Würzburg of being murderers of women and infants. In the end his practice of antiseptic hand-washing to prevent childbed fever was stopped, and the incidence of the disease rose to record levels.

Semmelweis became uncontrollably psychotic in his later years—most likely the result of syphilis or Alzheimer's—and was committed to an asylum, where he died of a wound infection in 1865, at the age of forty-seven. He had died of childbed fever.

The story of germs and their importance in disease would not be complete without discussing the work of another scientist, who shares with Pasteur the distinction of having founded medical microbiology. He was a quiet microbe hunter—as methodical as Pasteur was impulsive and as reserved as Pasteur was flamboyant—who did not care for Pasteur very much. His name was Robert Koch.

That Nasty Little German

Koch was born on December 11, 1843, in a small town in Germany. He studied medicine at the University of Göttingen and became a doctor in 1866. He interned at an insane asylum in Hamburg and then moved on to private practice, earning better than five dollars on a good day. But he was restless and frustrated. Too many of his patients died, and he could do little to help them.

"I hate this bluff that my practice is," he complained. "Mothers come to me crying—asking me to save their babies—and what can I do?—Grope . . . fumble . . . reassure them when there is no hope. How can I cure a disease when I do not even know what causes it, when the wisest doctor in Germany doesn't know?" (*Microbe Hunters*, by Paul deKruif).

Then, for his twenty-eighth birthday, his wife, Emmy, bought him a microscope to play with. It proved to be a truly historic gift. Much as

Leeuwenhoek had done two centuries earlier, he put everything he could find under the lenses of his microscope. His focus, however, was the causative agents of disease. More than any other scientist, including Pasteur, he established the concept that a specific microbe causes a specific disease—the one germ/one disease theory. In 1876 he isolated and identified the anthrax bacillus and demonstrated that it alone caused the blood of sheep, cows, and people to blacken with that often fatal disease. In 1882 he isolated and identified a slender rod-shaped bacterium and demonstrated that it alone caused the disease that has killed more humans than any other: tuberculosis. In 1883 he entered a race with Pasteur to isolate and identify the bacterium that caused cholera, an often fatal diarrheal disease of humans—entirely different from chicken cholera, discussed earlier—that still kills millions in India and other third-world countries. It was a race that he won.

Koch was a brilliant investigator, and in the laboratory, amid his culture flasks and dyes and slide preparations, he had no equal. To quote Stanley Wedberg (*Introduction to Microbiology*), former head of the Department of Bacteriology at the University of Connecticut, Koch "introduced order out of the laboratory chaos existing in the 1860s. Among his accomplishments were methods for placing microbes on glass slides and then staining them with various dyes to make them more visible under a microscope." This enabled scientists to better study and distinguish between microbes that were similar in size and shape. Koch also put together recipes to grow bacteria that were especially finicky in their eating habits. He was the first to photograph bacteria through a microscope. But his most enduring contribution to laboratory procedures was his invention of a method for growing microorganisms in pure culture. It is a technique used in every bacteriology lab today exactly as Koch developed it more than a hundred years ago. And it would never have happened were it not for a boiled potato.

In microbiology it is important to be able to grow germs pure, without other kinds of germs growing in the same culture vessel mixed in with them. Otherwise it becomes extremely difficult to prove that *this* particular germ causes *that* particular disease. But there are few places in nature where bacteria exist as pure, individual species. Expose a flask of beef broth to the air for ten seconds, and in less than a day it will be teeming with the offspring of a dozen different kinds of bacteria and molds.

Bacteriologists devoted themselves to the problem of growing organisms pure. According to Paul deKruif, in *Microbe Hunters*: "All manner of weird machines were being invented to try to keep different sorts of germs apart. Several microbe hunters devised apparatus so complicated that when they had finished building it they probably had already forgotten what they set out to invent it for. To keep stray germs of the air from falling into their bottles some heroic searchers did their inoculations in an actual rain of poisonous germicides!"

Then one day Koch happened to notice sitting on a table in his laboratory a sliced section of boiled potato. On its flat surface was a curious collection of colored droplets—one gray, another red, a third yellow—contamination in Technicolor.

As with Pasteur's chicken cholera vaccine, the discovery was serendipitous. And once again, chance favored the prepared mind. Koch proceeded to suspend the material from each droplet into a bit of water and look at it under the microscope. What he saw was a pure colony of bacteria in each droplet. Where a bacterium had landed on the potato from the air it multiplied into a droplet or colony of billions of identical bacteria. It grew pure.

The key lay not in the potato itself but in its solid surface—a concept so simple that it was elegant. Growth cultures had always been liquids—beef or chicken broth or blood serum. In a liquid, microbes mix. On a solid surface they stay in one place; they remain separate. And that made all the difference.

The potato was quickly replaced with other solid media more suitable to bacterial taste buds. An early substitute was gelatin mixed with a variety of goodies to induce bacterial growth. But gelatin is a liquid at human body temperature, and most microbes pathogenic to humans grow best at that temperature.

Enter Fanny Eilshemius, a laboratory technician in Koch's employ. In making her jams and jellies at home, she used a constituent of Japanese seaweed as a solidifying material. It was called agar-agar. She suggested this material to Koch, and he tried it. Agar-agar proved an ideal solidifying agent. It did not liquefy easily, with either heat or the enzymatic action of microbes. Agar-agar (now called agar) remains today the solidifying agent of choice for pure culture procedures. Unfortunately, Fanny Eilshemius did not receive her fair share of the credit for its discovery.

Koch's contributions to microbiology and the advancement of the germ theory of disease are legend. They rival those of the great Pasteur himself, who referred to Koch with passionate disfavor as "that nasty little German from Berlin." As with Pasteur, he had a research institution dedicated to him, the Koch Institute in Berlin, a prestigious center for microbial studies. He will be remembered again in Chapter 4, "The White Death," which deals with tuberculosis, a disease that marks both the height and depth of his remarkable career.

3

Magic Bullets

When a lot of remedies are suggested for a disease, that means it can't be cured.

— ANTON CHEKHOV

BY THE DAWN of the twentieth century vaccines against a number of deadly diseases had been discovered, and the methodology was well established. Aseptic and antiseptic procedures had greatly reduced the incidence of generalized infection, or sepsis, from surgery, injury, and childbirth. But these measures were preventive. Doctors were virtually powerless to *cure* disease. Once a person was afflicted, there was little the physician could do other than inject morphine for the pain and hope that the person's natural defenses would prevail. For many unfortunate sufferers they did not. Women who contracted puerperal fever still died of it. Wound infections were still fatal nearly as often as not. In fact, during World War II four out of every five fatalities were from wound infections rather than the wounds themselves. Tuberculosis was the number one killer among developed nations, including the United States. In essence infectious diseases were untreatable. But the Age of Antibiotics was on the horizon, an era in which doctors would build an arsenal of chemical weapons with which to combat Pasteur's "malignant microbes."

As of this writing, about 160 different antibiotics are on the market in the United States alone, with dozens more on the runway. It is difficult to keep count. Farmers treat their cows and hogs and chickens with a superabundance of antibiotics. Salmon and trout on fish farms get drugs in their water; honeybees, in their hives. A glass of milk may contain minute amounts of up to eighty different kinds. Antibiotic pesticides rain down on crops to the tune of three hundred thousand pounds (136,000 kilograms) a year. After having suffered through countless plagues over millennia, we embraced these magic bullets with uncommon passion, and the love affair goes on.

The First Chemotherapy

Paul Ehrlich was born the son of a successful German businessman on March 14, 1854. Although he did poorly in school, Ehrlich demonstrated a singular interest and aptitude in both chemistry and biology. At the age of eight he had the town pharmacist prepare cough drops according to a prescription he had put together himself.

Ehrlich attended medical school at Leipzig, where he graduated in 1878. His graduation thesis was on the application of dyes in staining bacteria, an interest he would return to in later years. Dyes had always been a valuable product in the textile industry, but in the late 1800s Robert Koch and other microbiologists had started using them to color bacteria as well. The use of appropriate stains and staining techniques in fact facilitated Koch's identification in 1882 of the bacillus that causes tuberculosis.

Shortly after that discovery Ehrlich began to work for Koch. He quickly improved the technique for staining the tubercle bacillus—one that, with slight modification, is used today, more than one hundred twenty years later. In 1886 he contracted the dreaded tuberculosis himself and retired to Egypt, where he hoped that rest and the favorable climate would cure him. Fortunately his case was a mild one, and he recovered.

Upon his return from Egypt in 1889, Ehrlich teamed up with two other bacteriologists, Emil von Behring, a fellow countryman, and Shibasaburo Kitasato of Japan. Over a three-year period they developed a cure for the horrid childhood killer diphtheria. The achievement won Behring the first Nobel Prize in Physiology or Medicine (1901) and Ehrlich a professorship at the University of Berlin. (Sadly, Behring and Ehrlich would part in anger after a quarrel.) Several years later the German government opened an institute for serum research, and Ehrlich was put in charge. The work was an extension of what he had done with Behring and Kitasato on diphtheria, and his continuing efforts in the field earned him a Nobel Prize in Physiology or Medicine seven years after Behring.

As is sometimes the case, Nobel Prize–winning work is not the crowning achievement in a person's career. Albert Einstein was awarded the Nobel in Physics for his explanation of a phenomenon called the photoelectric effect, yet his theories of relativity were far more dramatic and sweeping in scope, and were the substance of his unprecedented popularity. So it was with Paul Ehrlich. Despite his success with diphtheria and serum immunology, his grand vision for curing disease was through his stains, and it was in this area that he made his most enduring contribution. To quote Isaac Asimov in his *Biographical Encyclopedia of Science and Technology*:

> *Ehrlich reasoned that the value of a stain was that it colored some cells and not others; it colored bacteria, for instance, and made them stand out against a colorless background. Well, a stain could not color bacteria unless it combined with some substance in the bacterium and if it did that it would usually kill the bacterium. If a dye could be found that stained bacteria and not ordinary cells, it might represent a chemical that killed bacteria without harming human beings. Ehrlich would have, in effect, a "magic bullet" that could be taken into the body where it would seek out the parasites and destroy them.*

Ehrlich devoted the latter part of his life to this "magic bullet" concept, performing thousands of experiments over more than a dozen years. His patience and perseverance were incredible. More often than not there were no magic bullets, but occasionally his labors bore fruit. He discovered a dye, called trypan red, that cured a laboratory mouse infected with the often-fatal disease sleeping sickness, or trypanosomiasis. When tested on human sufferers, however, it did not work.

Ehrlich wondered about this. He believed that the action of trypan red could be attributed to a particular grouping of nitrogen atoms in the molecule. Arsenic belongs to the same chemical family as nitrogen but is distinctly more poisonous. Ehrlich decided to replace the nitrogen atoms in trypan red with arsenic. It was an inspiring concept: manipulate the structure of a molecule in small ways to alter its chemical properties and its action on living systems. Chemists in the years to follow would rely heavily on this approach in their struggle to find new chemicals to combat old diseases. Paul Ehrlich was their founding father.

Ehrlich certainly had his shortcomings. He was not an easy person to work for. He was argumentative in the extreme and ran his workshop more like a dictatorship than a democracy. He chain-smoked cigars and could down a pint of ale with the best of them. But he was a gifted and tireless experimenter. He manipulated the trypan red molecule in countless ways, removing a nitrogen here, adding an arsenic there, replacing one side chain, modifying another. In 1907, on his 606th manipulation, he came up with dihydroxydiamino-arsenobenzene hydrochloride. It did not work very well against the bug that caused sleeping sickness, and Ehrlich passed over it, garnering his Nobel in the meantime.

Two years later a new assistant of Ehrlich's happened to test "606" on the organism that causes syphilis—a corkscrew-shaped bacterium called a *spirochete*. (Spirochetes also cause the tick-borne Lyme disease, discussed in Chapter 5, "New Kids on the Block.") It was very effective in killing the microorganism. Ehrlich immediately seized on the finding. Syphilis was a much more dreaded disease than sleeping sickness, infecting many famous and infamous people: King Henry VIII of England, Louis XIV of France, Peter the Great, Napoléon Bonaparte, George Armstrong Custer, "Wild Bill" Hickok, Abraham Lincoln's wife, Winston Churchill's father, Al Capone, and about half a million Americans today. It can damage internal organs, including the circulatory and nervous systems, and can lead to seizures, personality changes, mental debilitation, heart disease, and death.

In 1910, after clinical testing of 606—which he named *salvarsan*—Ehrlich announced his discovery to the world. Although salvarsan was an effective treatment for syphilis, it was poisonous to the human body as well. Unless dosages were followed carefully, the patient could experience fatal toxicity. As a result, Ehrlich was attacked by some doctors as a quack and a murderer. These accusations affected him deeply, leading to alcohol

abuse, and contributed to his premature death in 1915. But the accusations were unfair. Salvarsan cured many more lives than it killed—and from the vantage point of historical perspective Ehrlich is regarded as one of the great benefactors of humankind. Trypan red and salvarsan mark the beginning of the science and medical procedure called *chemotherapy*, a term coined by Ehrlich.

The First Antibiotic

René Dubos was born in a small village near Paris on February 20, 1901. His formal education as a child was poor, often in cold and dark one-room schoolhouses with inadequately trained teachers. But René had a passion for reading and learning, and largely he was self-taught.

Most important, however, he was fascinated with humus, a rich mix of soil and decomposing organic matter. Dubos wondered how microbes broke down the organic matter—mainly the bodies of bugs and the cellulose of leaves and twigs—and formed the growth medium so cherished by farmers around the world. He studied soil microbiology at the French National College of Agriculture.

In 1924 he attended a conference in Rome on soil science. There he met the Russian-born scientist Selman Waksman, who was a world authority on soil microbiology. Waksman was impressed with Dubos and offered him a job in his laboratory at the Agricultural College of Rutgers in New Brunswick, New Jersey. Dubos accepted the offer and also enrolled in courses toward an advanced degree in bacteriology. The training he received in soil microbiology, both at the college and in Waksman's laboratory, would later prove invaluable. When it came time for his doctoral degree, Dubos chose to do research on microorganisms that break down cellulose in soil—an old favorite of his. He succeeded in isolating a soil bacterium that was capable of dissolving paper, a cellulose-based substance.

After completing his thesis, Dubos applied for a National Research Council fellowship but was turned down because he was not an American citizen. In the margin of the rejection letter, however, was a suggestion from a kindly secretary advising him to seek help from Dr. Alexis Carrel, a fellow Frenchman working at the renowned Rockefeller Institute in New York City. It was advice that would profoundly change Dubos's life and the course of history.

Dubos went to the Rockefeller to see the eminent French vascular surgeon. Dr. Carrel was sympathetic and understanding but had nothing to offer Dubos. He was, after all, a surgeon, not a soil microbiologist. Over lunch he introduced Dubos to a fellow worker at the institute, a Canadian-born bacteriologist by the name of Oswald Avery. Dubos discussed his work on soil bacteria and cellulose decomposition with Avery, who was deeply interested. Avery was doing research of his own on a particular bacterium that caused pneumonia in humans—*Streptococcus pneumoniae*, or pneumococcus. When grown in an artificial medium, colonies of pneumococcus took two distinctly different forms: smooth-edged (S-form) and rough-edged (R-form). S-form pneumococcus was pathogenic and caused pneumonia; R-form did not. On a microscopic level S-form pneumococci were surrounded by a polysaccharide capsule; R-forms were not. It was the capsule surrounding the bacteria that made them pathogenic. Avery reasoned that if a chemical that destroyed the polysaccharide capsule could be found, an effective treatment for pneumococcal pneumonia could be gotten. He also knew that cellulose is a polysaccharide—not unlike the capsule surrounding his S-form bacteria. If Dubos had found a microbe in his beloved humus that digested cellulose, might he not also find one that could digest capsular polysaccharide?

Avery concluded their lunchtime chat by offering Dubos a job in his laboratory. It was the beginning of a relationship that lasted twenty years and was extremely productive on both sides. Their enduring collaboration would help Avery make one of the most significant discoveries in all of science: that DNA is the hereditary material. It founded the discipline of modern genetics.

Working in Avery's lab, Dubos developed a culture medium in which the capsular polysaccharide was the sole source of food and then inoculated different soil and sewage microbes (including his paper-digesting bacterium) into these cultures. He had no success. The microbes did not digest the polysaccharide. Then Dubos remembered the cranberry bogs, a swampy region in New Jersey not far from Rutgers University, where he had worked for several years with Dr. Waksman. Among the cranberries and cattails that grew there, a gummy polysaccharide collected. At times the collection thinned. Something in the bogs had to be decomposing it.

Dubos wrote to Waksman for a sample of soil from the cranberry bogs. Immediately upon receiving it he began inoculating his culture tubes

with suspensions of cranberry-bog-soil microbes. For the first time the microorganisms began to grow, devouring the capsular polysaccharide as if it were a pepperoni pizza. Something was producing an enzyme that digested the capsule. Dubos was feverish with excitement. In a short time he was able to isolate the "something" in pure culture—a previously unknown bacterium that he appropriately dubbed the Cranberry Bog Bacillus (CBB).

Dubos did not immediately report his work to Avery, who had begun his summer vacation. Instead he concentrated his efforts on isolating the stuff responsible for digesting the polysaccharide capsule. After a week or two he had a crude extract of the CBB enzyme.

The next step was to determine if the enzyme had any clinical effect in either preventing or curing pneumococcal pneumonia in laboratory animals. Throughout the summer of 1929 Dubos injected mice with the deadly bacterium and then with the CBB extract. It worked. In trial after trial mice that were injected with the enzyme and then with a fatal dose of pneumococcus showed no signs of illness.

Dubos decided it was time to notify Avery. The senior scientist cut his summer vacation short, returning quickly to the Rockefeller. Additional experiments were performed and improvements made under Avery's guidance. Precise dosages of the enzyme and a timetable for their use were established. Then, in 1930 in the journal *Science*, they announced their discovery to the world.

Their achievement was received by both the lay and scientific communities with great enthusiasm. For the first time in history man had discovered and isolated a substance produced in one microorganism that would counteract the disease-causing effects of another. Fifteen years later Selman Waksman, Dubos's mentor at Rutgers, would define such chemicals; he would call them *antibiotics*.*

---

*Today the term *antibiotic* is used more broadly to include semisynthetic and fully synthetic compounds, dulling the distinction between antibiotics and chemotherapies. In fact, this dulling creates a legitimate argument. Antibiotics are considered to be useful against bacteria but not viruses. However, if synthetic drugs are being called antibiotics, why can't *antivirals*—which are synthesized—such as acyclovir (used to treat chicken pox, shingles, and the herpes complex) or AZT (used to treat AIDS) be called antibiotics? Perhaps they can. But even so, there are only about half a dozen viral infections that are treatable with these agents, and they do not include the most common ones, such as the common cold or influenza. In this book, antibiotics will be viewed as *antibacterials*.

Amid growing excitement and popularity, Dubos and Avery continued their work on the CBB enzyme, testing it not only in mice but in rats, rabbits, and monkeys as well. The results were invariably positive. It was time to test the enzyme in humans. The world eagerly awaited the first trials. Dubos would later say, "Emotionally, this was my greatest hour in science!"

But the trials never happened, and Dubos's greatest hour in science turned into his greatest disappointment. In another part of the world a rival antibacterial agent had just been discovered, one that made the Cranberry Bog Bacillus enzyme clinically redundant. The rival discovery—called Prontosil—would prove both safer and more effective than the CBB enzyme in treating particular bacterial infections.

Dubos would experience bitter disappointment in his professional life a second time, ten years later. Still working at the Rockefeller and with soil microbes, he would discover a new bacterium, *Bacillus brevis*, which produced a substance that killed Gram-positive bacteria—including the deadly pneumococcus, staphylococcus, and streptococcus. (Bacteria are classified as Gram-positive or Gram-negative based on the way they respond to a certain staining technique.) Dubos called it, aptly, *gramicidin*. It was an incredibly effective antibiotic. One microgram of gramicidin would protect a mouse from a thousand times the fatal dose of pneumococcus. Drug companies became intensely interested in its structure and pharmacology. It was tested exhaustively in different laboratory animals. Sadly it was found to be poisonous to the host organism. It destroyed red blood cells and caused serious kidney damage. Although it might still have value as a topical salve or cream, it would never be used to cure serious systemic infections.

Despite his seeming failures, Dubos's lifelong dedication and contribution to medicine cannot be overstated. He is indeed the father of antibiotics and is regarded as one of the giants in the modern era of medicine. His work was the inspiration that would lead Waksman to discover streptomycin and Florey and Chain to rediscover penicillin.

But the first of the miracle drugs to be used commercially was neither of these.

The First Wonder Drug

For the story of Prontosil we must cross the Atlantic and travel back in time to 1895, where in the small town of Lagów, Germany (now Poland),

Gerhard Johannes Domagk was born. After a carefree and comfortable childhood Domagk enrolled at the University of Kiel Medical School. Shortly thereafter World War I broke out in Europe, and Domagk, with youthful patriotism, enlisted with several of his classmates. He was trained as a medical assistant and sent to field hospitals on the eastern front to tend to the wounded soldiers. It was there that his patriotic idealism flagged and he became aware of the brutality and senselessness of war. He also witnessed the horrors of infection that had haunted Pasteur and Lister and Semmelweis. In some wards soldiers died as often from wound infection as from injury. These included the ubiquitous strep and staph infections, which were usually fatal if they got into the bloodstream, and gangrene, which produced a foul-smelling gas that bubbled from blackened, putrefying flesh and caused death from toxemia if the infected part was not amputated. The sights that Domagk saw in the field hospitals would both torment and inspire him for the rest of his life.

After the war ended, Domagk returned to medical school. Money was scarce and times were difficult in postwar Germany. Domagk had little to eat or wear and often went hungry and cold. But he had a singular dedication. He once fainted in class from hunger and overwork.

Domagk earned his medical degree in 1921 and worked as a junior doctor at the City Hospital in Kiel. Two years later he transferred to the Pathological Institute of Greifswald University, where he did important research on the human immune system. He made an important discovery: bacteria that were damaged in some way were more readily destroyed by the body's immune system than healthy bacteria. It was an observation that would prove pivotal in his later work.

The turning point of Domagk's career came in 1927 when, at the age of thirty-one, he was asked to work for the Bayer company of I. G. Farbenindustrie, the great German dye firm. The president of Bayer, Carl Duisberg, was a staunch advocate of chemotherapy, the medical treatment against infection popularized by Paul Ehrlich. But chemotherapy was not highly regarded by the medical community. The thought of swallowing arsenic or iodine or cyanide was, to say the least, repulsive. Even the great Robert Koch had frowned on chemotherapy as a feasible treatment.

I. G. Farbenindustrie was, however, a chemical research think tank employing some of the world's greatest chemists to discover new and better products. In the late 1800s chemists at Bayer, its pharmaceutical division, discovered the wonder drug for pain, aspirin. In 1916 they discovered Germanin, the first treatment in history for sleeping sickness. They also discovered a drug that replaced quinine as the standard antimalarial treatment.

These successes convinced Duisberg that chemotherapy held much promise. Domagk attracted his attention because of the work he had done on the action of the human immune system on bacterial infections.

At Bayer, Domagk focused his efforts on diseases caused by streptococcus: the dreaded childbed fever; the often fatal scarlet fever; rheumatic fever, which damaged the heart and kidneys; and blood poisoning, which was always fatal. (In Chapter 5, "New Kids on the Block," strep infections will be discussed as a growing threat.)

Domagk was not immediately successful. Working with a brilliant chemist, Josef Klarer, he tested many hundreds of compounds for antistreptococcal properties between 1927 and 1932. Five days before Christmas in 1932, he tested an orange-red crystal that had had no success in killing streptococcus in a test tube, injecting it into mice that had been given a fatal dose of strep. His colleagues, who had little confidence in Domagk's work and even less in the concept of chemotherapy, were astonished when all the injected mice lived—in fact showed no signs of illness at all. After five long years of failure, Domagk too could not believe his eyes. "We stood there astounded . . . as if we had suffered an electric shock."

The chemical was given the trade name Prontosil. It was a member of the sulfonamides, a group of compounds distinguished by their ring structure and sulfur atom attached to the ring. To his colleagues, who had not understood why he thought a chemical that had failed to kill the germ in a test tube would do so inside a mouse, Domagk could have explained that Prontosil worked by damaging bacterial cells, which could then be destroyed more easily by the body's immune system. Prontosil proved extremely effective in treating not only strep but many Gram-positive infections, including staph and gas gangrene, the infection that had haunted Domagk since his days at the battlefront hospitals during World War I. In 1932 it saved the life of his young daughter, Hildegarde, who had been infected by strep after being pricked by a needle, and in 1936 it saved the life of Franklin Delano Roosevelt Jr., son of the president of the United States. During World War II it saved the lives of thousands of wounded

German soldiers. Although it had occasional serious side effects, Prontosil was without question the first of the wonder drugs.

Shortly after its discovery, two French doctors tinkered with the sulfonamide molecule, changing it subtly. What they came up with was a compound much simpler to put together, even more effective, and preparable in a form that could be taken orally. It was called *sulfanilamide*. In subsequent years more than thirteen hundred derivatives of sulfanilamide have been synthesized for use as chemotherapies. Collectively they are known as the *sulfa drugs*, and they were indeed a miracle. For the first time in history a tablet or an injection could be given to fight infection, to alleviate suffering, and to prevent death.

For his discovery of Prontosil, Domagk was awarded the Nobel Prize in Physiology or Medicine in 1939. There was a problem, however. Four years earlier another German, Carl von Ossietzky, had been awarded the Nobel Prize for Peace. Ossietzky was a pacifist who had publicly denounced the activities of the Third Reich. Ossietzky was imprisoned in a concentration camp, where he died of tuberculosis in 1938. The entire incident proved an international embarrassment to Hitler and his war machine. Against this backdrop Domagk was ordered to refuse the Nobel Prize. Eight years later, with the end of World War II and the demise of Hitler and the Third Reich, Domagk would finally accept his award in Stockholm, Sweden.

Prontosil was the first of the miracle drugs to be marketed successfully, but it was not the first to be discovered. Four years before Prontosil came on the scene, a common bread mold was killing bacteria in a petri dish in a small and cluttered laboratory in England.

The Miracle Mold

Alexander Fleming was born on August 6, 1881, in Lochfield, Scotland, one of eight children. At the age of thirteen he left Scotland for England with his brothers in search of better educational and career opportunities. For four years he worked as a shipping clerk. An inheritance left to him by an uncle in 1901 enabled Fleming to enter medical school at St. Mary's Hospital in London. Five years later he received his medical license and joined the Inoculation Department of St. Mary's (now the Wright-Fleming Institute), where he worked until his death, in 1955, of a heart attack. At the department he worked under the supervision of the brilliant Dr. Almroth Wright. Wright was a confirmed believer in immunotherapy for the treatment of disease and did not put much stock in antibacterial chemicals such as salvarsan—still widely used at the time in the treatment of syphilis.

During World War I, Fleming served in the Royal Army Medical Corps, specializing in the treatment of wounds with antiseptics. Like Domagk, he was horrified by the brutality of war and its attendant suffering and death.

After the war, Fleming became assistant director of the Inoculation Department at St. Mary's. He discovered a substance in bodily secretions that destroyed bacterial cells. He called it *lysozyme*. Unfortunately, it was effective only against nonpathogenic bacteria. Its discovery, however, stimulated Fleming's interest in the search for a substance that would selectively destroy pathogenic bacteria.

He found what he was looking for in 1928, although it was indeed a serendipitous discovery. By nature Fleming was rather untidy in his work habits. He would leave old and discarded bacterial cultures lying around for weeks before disposing of them. On one occasion a contaminant from the air happened to get into one of these cultures—a petri dish on which colonies of staphylococcus were peppered. The contaminant grew into a wrinkled and fuzzy green blob the size of a bottle cap. Around the blob there was no staph.

Fleming recognized the green fuzz immediately as *Penicillium*, a mold commonly found on spoiling bread and fruit. The clear area surrounding the mold intrigued him, and as with Pasteur and his birds that had recovered from chicken cholera and Koch with his slice of boiled potato that had become contaminated, accident would lead to important discovery. The clear area around the penicillium was a zone of inhibited growth; the mold was secreting a substance that prevented the staph from multiplying. Fleming called this substance "mould juice," later renaming it *penicillin*. He immediately realized the potential of his discovery as a weapon against bacterial infection. If a germ could not multiply, it could not cause disease.

Penicillin was found to be effective against not only staph germs but a wide spectrum of pathogens, including those that cause strep infections, gonorrhea, syphilis, and gas gangrene. (It would replace salvarsan for the treatment of syphilis.) But there was a terrible downside. Mould juice proved to be very unstable, rapidly losing its antibacterial activity. It was also extremely difficult to purify. Fleming was not a chemist and did not have the ability to solve these problems, without which penicillin was of no practical use. He received little encouragement or support from Dr. Wright. This was unfortunate, for it delayed the useful preparation of what many consider to be medical science's greatest contribution to humanity.

Ten years later two researchers working at Oxford, the Australian-born pathologist Howard Florey and the German biochemist Ernst Chain, while investigating antimicrobial agents, uncovered Fleming's paper on penicillin. Using a technique called *lyophilization*, or freeze-drying (similar to the procedure used today to prepare instant coffee), they successfully isolated the drug in pure form, which was a million times more active than Fleming's mould juice. They were also able to increase its stability.

With a purified and relatively stable form of penicillin, Florey and Chain proceeded to test laboratory animals. In 1940 they published the results of their successful treatment of infected white mice. They were assisted by Norman Heatley, a friend and colleague of Florey's at Oxford.

Florey decided to test penicillin on a human volunteer in early 1941. He chose Albert Alexander, a forty-three-year-old police constable who had been scratched near the mouth by a rose thorn. According to Edwin Kiester Jr. in his article "A Curiosity Turned into the First Silver Bullet Against Death," in the November 1990 issue of *Smithsonian*: "The simple wound had developed both staphylococcal and streptococcal infections. Alexander had multiple abscesses of the head and face; his lungs were infected; one eye had been removed. He was in great pain and the only hope was for a merciful death."

Then penicillin was administered. In less than a day Alexander's fever dropped and he began to improve. But there was not enough penicillin to last for more than a few days. It would not be enough to cure Alexander's massive infection, unless . . . . It was known that much of penicillin passed through the body unchanged and was rapidly excreted in the urine. More than half of a dose could be recovered in this way. Each day the policeman's urine was collected, and then penicillin was separated from it and reused. (This was also done later on, with wounded soldiers being given penicillin.) But with each separation some penicillin was lost. After five days Alexander's fever had disappeared, his appetite had returned, and the infection that had taken an eye and nearly his life was all but gone. Then the penicillin ran out. As Kiester retells it, "Alexander clung to life gamely for another month. But finally, after being on the brink of recovery, he died."

Though the patient died, the operation was a clear-cut success. The team knew that penicillin could be used to defeat human infection—if only they had enough of it. Toward this end the United States, with its booming pharmaceutical industry, would join forces with its overseas ally.

The first truly successful treatment of a human being with penicillin happened in the spring of 1942. Anne Miller was a patient at New Haven Hospital in Connecticut. She had contracted a streptococcal infection from her son, who had recently recovered from a bout with strep throat. Her bloodstream was brimming with the bacteria, and she had developed an inflammation in the large blood vessels in her pelvis and thighs. Her temperature had reached nearly 107°F (42°C); she was delirious. Doctors had given her blood transfusions, sulfa drugs, and even rattlesnake serum, to no avail. There was no hope. Anne Miller would die. Her brother-in-law remarked at her bedside, "When you turned away . . . for a minute, you didn't know if she'd be alive when you looked back."

Then on Saturday, March 14, a small brown bottle in a brown bag arrived from England with the instructions "Don't drop it on the floor." The bottle contained about a teaspoonful of penicillin. By 3:30 that afternoon Anne Miller received her first injection of the drug. She received subsequent injections every four hours, through the night—a total of about thirty-five thousand units. (Today a dose of one million units is commonplace.) By 9:00 A.M. Sunday her temperature was normal for the first time in four weeks, and all her vital signs were stable. By Sunday afternoon she was sitting up in bed acting as if she had never been ill. According to Dr. Thomas Sappington, her attending physician, "Nothing in my whole experience has ever compared to that. Nothing like it had ever happened before." (Anne Miller died on May 27, 1999, in Salisbury, Connecticut, at the age of ninety. Penicillin extended her life fifty-seven years.)

In the meantime, World War II had begun. Penicillin saved the lives of many thousands of Allied soldiers during the war and of millions of civilians in subsequent years. It was also remarkably nontoxic to human tissue.

Fleming received many honorary degrees and awards for his discovery of penicillin. In 1944 both he and Florey were knighted, and in 1945 they received, along with Chain, the Nobel Prize in Physiology or Medicine. In succeeding years Fleming would become an international celebrity; film star Marlene Dietrich once cooked dinner for him at a private party, just so she could meet the man who had saved the lives of countless soldiers in the field hospitals at the European front, where she had entertained the GIs. Florey and his group at Oxford would continue to do groundbreaking work with antibiotics. Chain, sadly, would leave Oxford bitter and resentful, believing that he had never received proper credit for his work on penicillin and that the American pharmaceutical companies had exploited him. (Fleming himself never collected royalties on penicillin, but American chemical firms collected $100,000 and presented it to him as a gift of gratitude. He declined acceptance personally, using the money instead for research at St. Marys.)

Today the "penicillins" represent a diverse group of more than fifty chemically related antibiotics, developed over the years from more than ten thousand variants. A similar chemical compound, also derived from a mold, was cephalosporin, which also has a large family of relatives. The vast majority of antibiotics are either penicillins or cephalosporins. Some are natural, while others are partly or fully synthetic. Despite their differences, they all have a common chemistry and modality.

Fleming remains one of the great heroes of modern medicine. According to André Maurois, a Fleming biographer, "No man, except Einstein in another field, and before him Pasteur, has had a more profound influence on the contemporary history of the human race." In the book *Medicine's 10 Greatest Discoveries*, Meyer Friedman and Gerald Friedland, along with a concensus of medical doctors and physicians, list Fleming's synthesis of penicillin, along with Jenner's cowpox vaccine. Fleming would also inspire in no small way another hero of modern medicine, the discoverer of the next miracle drug, streptomycin. It did not come from a mold in the air but from the "good earth."

A Miracle from the Soil

Although many people must be mentioned in the story of streptomycin, it is essentially a tale of two scientists—one who was recognized for his contribution and awarded the highest prize in his field and one who was not.

The Father of Soil Microbiology

Zolman Abraham Waksman was born on July 8, 1888, in the Russian Ukraine. He had a happy childhood despite the fact that, being a Jew in czarist Russia, he suffered ridicule and persecution. He came from a poor family and had to earn money by tutoring to pay for teachers to advance his own education. Above all, he loved the land; he had a passion for it. In his autobiography, *My Life with the Microbes*, he said, "The odour of the black soil so filled my lungs that I was never able to forget it." The study of the soil would become his life's work.

In 1910 Waksman's mother died. The winds of war were stirring in Europe, and revolution was imminent in his own country. He decided to leave Russia for America, where the future was a great deal more promising.

Waksman landed at Philadelphia on November 2, 1910, and went to live on a farm in New Jersey with his cousin. He enrolled in the Agricultural College at Rutgers, where he studied soil microbiology, and graduated in 1915 with a bachelor of science degree. That year he Americanized his name to Selman Waksman and married the sister of his best friend. Less than a year later he added a master's degree to his list of achievements.

Armed with his degrees, he traveled to the Department of Agriculture in Washington, D.C., where he worked and studied for several years, and got a Ph.D. in biochemistry. Now thirty-one, he returned to Rutgers, where he taught soil microbiology and did groundbreaking research that identified many previously unknown bacteria and molds in the soil. One organism in particular, which he named *Actinomyces griseus*, would assume great importance in his later work.

In 1939 Waksman—by then a full professor and a world authority on soil science since the 1927 publication of his seminal text *Principles of Soil Microbiology*—attended the Third International Congress of Microbiology in New York City. One of the keynote speakers was Alexander Fleming. Waksman was transfixed by Fleming's speech about a common bread mold called penicillin. If Fleming could find a miracle microbe in the air, he could find one in the soil. From that moment he would devote himself not to the study of soil microbes per se but to their importance in developing agents against disease—in particular, diseases caused by Gram-negative bacteria. These were the pathogens that were resistant to all the previously developed antibiotics and chemotherapies: Prontosil, penicillin, and the ill-fated gramicidin and Cranberry Bog Bacillus enzyme. They included *E. coli* (a normal resident of the human colon), *Salmonella*, *Shigella*, and *V. cholerae* (the agent of cholera). They caused severe diarrhea, dysentery, bladder and kidney infections, abscesses in organs of the digestive system, and peritonitis, for starters. Collectively they killed millions of people each year.

Rutgers, meanwhile, through its association with Waksman, had been transformed from a simple agricultural college to a world-famous institution. It became a magnet school, attracting some of the most gifted and dedicated students and providing Waksman with the quality personnel he needed.

In 1940 Waksman's lab isolated a microorganism from the soil with distinctly antibacterial properties. It was an organism he was very familiar with—the funguslike actinomyces, which appeared as fuzzy colonies on solid media. One particular strain produced a powerful antibacterial substance, which he called *actinomycin*. With great expectation Waksman tested actinomycin on a group of infected laboratory mice. They all died within twenty-four to forty-eight hours—not from bacterial infection but from actinomycin. It was too toxic ever to be useful as an antibiotic.

A year later an assistant to Waksman isolated another actinomycete, *Streptomyces lavendulae*, which grew in pretty lavender colonies and had more powerful antibacterial properties than actinomycin, especially against the Gram-negatives. The active ingredient was isolated and called *streptothricin*. It was tested on mice and then cattle that had fatal infections. The results were dramatic. Streptothricin cured all the animals and did not harm them—at first. Unfortunately it had a delayed toxicity, which poisoned the kidneys and killed the animals weeks and even months later. Alas, streptothricin would find no practical use as an antibiotic either.

Then, in 1943, a young man came to Rutgers in search of his doctorate.

The Father of Streptomycin

Albert Schatz was born on February 2, 1920, in Norwich, Connecticut. His father was a farmer, and like Waksman, he had cultivated a love for the earth. He majored in soil chemistry as an undergraduate and came to Rutgers to get his Ph.D. in soil microbiology. He was not particularly interested in the investigation of microbes for antibacterial properties, but it was Waksman's passion, and he agreed to pursue it. Once into the search, however, Schatz became obsessed. According to Dr. Frank Ryan in *The Forgotten Plague*, Schatz worked in the lab from five in the morning until midnight or later, often eating and sleeping there as well. Schatz would say in an interview with Dr. Ryan, "I worked this intensively for several reasons. First I was fascinated by what I was doing; it intrigued me to no end. Secondly,

I fully realized how important it would be to find antibiotics effective in treating diseases caused by Gram-negative bacteria and even more so tuberculosis," which gives a variable and uninformative Gram stain.

After just three and a half months of sifting through thousands of soil bacteria, Schatz hit the jackpot. It was—what else?—an actinomycete. On agar it produced fuzzy gray colonies. It was *Actinomyces griseus* (subsequently renamed by Waksman *Streptomyces griseus*), the same organism that Waksman had discovered two dozen years earlier! Its antibacterial properties were amazing. It produced a substance significantly more effective than streptothricin in killing bacteria, Gram-positive *and* Gram-negative. When tested on animals, it showed little to no toxicity. (Subsequent testing would show that it caused deafness, dizziness, or tinnitus in about 10 percent of human recipients when given in high doses.) Waksman called it *streptomycin* and announced its discovery to the world in January 1944. It was also the first effective antibiotic against tuberculosis, a disease so feared that, of all the people working in Waksman's employ, only Schatz was willing to handle the microbe that caused it (see Chapter 4, "The White Death").

Streptomycin, behind Prontosil and penicillin, became the third of the world's great wonder drugs. For his achievement Selman Waksman was rewarded with his picture on the cover of the November 7, 1949, issue of *Time* and the Nobel Prize in Physiology or Medicine in 1952. Albert Schatz, the discoverer of streptomycin, was overlooked.

Awarding the Nobel to Waksman alone was indeed an injustice. That Waksman deserved the award was without question. Even if streptomycin had not been discovered, he could have gotten the Nobel for a lifetime of achievement in the field of soil microbiology. He wrote twenty-eight books and more than five hundred papers on the subject. He discovered and named more than a dozen different kinds of bacteria, including the genus *Streptomyces*, which produces more than half of the natural antibiotics on the market today. He was the architect of the program at Rutgers that systematically searched the soil for antibacterial agents.

But the discovery of streptomycin was Schatz's. The records list Waksman and Schatz as codiscoverers, which is only fair, but it was Schatz who first noticed its antibiotic properties, who isolated the organism producing it, who extracted, purified, and concentrated it. It was Schatz who ate and slept in the laboratory, testing and retesting the drug against an army of pathogens. The breakthrough was all Schatz's.

Why the Nobel committee did not include Schatz as a corecipient is unclear. Several years earlier Schatz had engaged in a bitter legal battle with Waksman regarding patent rights and subsequent royalties for the worldwide manufacture of streptomycin. The suit was settled out of court, and Schatz was awarded an initial payment of $125,000 and a share of the royalties for sale of the drug. But in retrospect this may have been a Pyrrhic victory. The scientific community had been shocked to its foundation by the audacity of a laboratory worker bringing legal suit against his mentor—especially one as well respected and world renowned as Dr. Waksman. It caused Waksman great public embarrassment and anguish. Perhaps the committee had not forgotten this. In any event, Schatz would never again work in a top-grade research laboratory. And he would not share in a prize that was awarded for the discovery of an antibiotic that he had discovered!

In his reception speech at the award ceremonies in Stockholm, Waksman would never mention the critical role that Albert Schatz had played in the whole streptomycin story. It was a sad and undeserved ending to what should have been a brilliant and enduring career.

Back to the Future

The war on disease was over! Antimicrobial drugs had won. Prontosil, penicillin, and streptomycin were followed by more powerful drugs with greater ability to wipe out pathogens. Laurie Garrett, in her encyclopedic work *The Coming Plague*, says: "By 1965 more than 25,000 different antibiotic products had been developed; physicians and scientists felt that bacterial diseases, and the microbes responsible, were no longer of great concern or of research interest."

Twenty-nine years later Rachel Nowak, in an article in *Science*, would write, "Childbirth is a gamble with death. Dental surgery potentially disabling. Even a facial boil can end in a trip to the morgue." Alexander Tomasz, microbiologist at Rockefeller University, recently confessed that we are on the verge of a medical nightmare that would turn back the clock to the days before antibiotics, when a paper cut or a skinned knee could lead to fatal infection. In U.S. hospitals, deaths from sepsis have increased sevenfold in the last twenty years. Deaths from infectious disease are up 58 percent since 1980. Yet there are more antibiotics on the market today than there ever have been. Why have infections, once again, become untreatable?

Resistance

The answer, in a word, is *resistance*. Microbes are finding ways to counteract or neutralize the effects of antibiotics, rendering them useless.
Despite the 160 or more on today's market, they are variations of only sixteen basic compounds and half a dozen modes of action. The germs have
found ways to foil these modes of action. They are the ultimate survivors.
Take penicillin for example. It works by inactivating an enzyme that bacteria need to make their cell wall. Without cell walls, bacteria cannot multiply and cause infection. They have developed resistance to penicillin by
breaking it down before it can inactivate the cell-wall-making enzyme or
by making a new enzyme that the penicillin cannot recognize. It took bacteria two years to develop penicillin resistance. The miracle drug came into
wide use in 1944, and the first resistant pathogens were reported in 1946.
By the late 1950s penicillin resistance was widespread. "Today," says
Madeline Drexler in *Secret Agents*, "just under 100 percent of *Staphylococcus aureus* are penicillin-resistant. And that's just the beginning."

Microbes have found ways of besting the other antibiotics as well.
Every germ has drug-resistant versions. The terrifying part is that some of
them have developed resistance to every known antibiotic. They are untreatable! Presently these untreatables are restricted to a group of bacteria called
enterococcus. It is not a very common group and does its infecting oppor-
tunistically, primarily in hospitals among the sick and elderly—people with
compromised immune systems. It causes urinary tract and wound infections and occasionally blood poisoning and meningitis, where it is quickly
fatal. Dr. Cynthia Gilbert, an infectious-disease specialist at the Veterans
Affairs Medical Center in Washington, experienced the frustration of such
untreatable infection. In 1993 she was treating a fifty-seven-year-old kidney patient who had developed an enterococcal blood infection. For nine
months Dr. Gilbert tried every antibiotic that was out there, individually
and in combination, orally and intravenously. Some would work for a while,
but then the infection would come roaring back. The patient eventually
died of a massive infection of the blood and heart. Today, about 20 percent
of enterococcal infections are totally drug resistant, and they kill thousands
of people every year.

Untreatable enterococcus is bad enough, but it is not a common agent
of infection outside of hospitals. Pneumococcus and staphylococcus are.

Hundreds of thousands of people get pneumococcal pneumonia in the United States alone every year. It also causes very serious wound infections and meningitis. It is responsible for perhaps half of the twenty-four million cases of earache in children, according to pediatricians. *Staphyloccus aureus* is the most common cause of skin, wound, and blood infections. It infects nine million Americans each year according to the CDC. Penicillin, once an effective antibiotic against staph, is now useless. Many strains of pneumococcus require dosages of penicillin more than a thousand times the original. Most frightening, however, is the fact that certain strains of pneumococcus and half the strains of *S. aureus* respond to only one antibiotic—vancomycin. And that response is eroding away. In May 1996 a Japanese baby developed a severe *S. aureus* infection. He was unsuccessfully treated with vancomycin. The infection was finally extinguished with a combination of vancomycin and the experimental drug Synercid. There have been other, similar cases, since. What happens when vancomycin and/or other drugs all fail to do the job? A lot of people will die. "You can die of a boil if there is no way to treat it," says one bacteriologist.

The future is indeed foreboding. In 1992 a British researcher demonstrated that vancomycin resistance can travel from enterococcus to staphylococcus. The finding was so frightening that the researcher immediately destroyed his entire stock of vancomycin-resistant staph. But the terrifying potential for disaster remains. In hospitals enterococcus and staphylococcus often share living quarters on wound bandages.

But how does resistance "travel" from one microbe to another?

Sex. Resistance is a genetic trait carried in the hereditary material of a particular microorganism. The exchange or transfer of this material among members of a population is called *sex*. The term has a rather limited application for humans and most other animals and plants. It is the uniting of two cells, a sperm and an egg, for the purpose of forming a new mix of genetic material, new combinations of traits, and greater variety among organisms within the population. For bacteria, sex is a much broader mechanism. Bacteria are truly promiscuous creatures, readily exchanging genetic material with other bacterial cells. And gene-swapping occurs across very wide taxonomic boundaries. Bacteria are not at all selective in choosing a sex partner.

The methods by which they transfer genetic material vary. Snippets of their regular DNA—that which makes up their single chromosome—can be transferred from one bacterium to another. The process is called *transformation*. Larger amounts of DNA can be transferred by a more intimate union of two bacteria in a process called *conjugation*. This method is more common than transformation and involves not chromosomal DNA but a separate, smaller piece of genetic material called a *plasmid*. Drug-resistant traits are more often carried in plasmids than in the chromosome itself. Cholera-causing bacteria picked up drug resistance to tetracycline from a plasmid in *E. coli*, a normal, harmless resident of the human gut.

Even more free-spirited than plasmids are things called "jumping genes," more formally known as *transposons*. They are mobile bits of DNA that move with relative ease among a population of bacteria, sharing traits which are likely to include resistance.

Viruses that attack bacteria (called *bacteriophages*) can also act as vehicles of genetic-material transfer, a process called *transduction*. To do their damage, viruses must get inside the bacterial cells, link their own genetic material with the bacteria's, multiply, and then break free. Viruses may carry drug-resistant genes from one bacterium to another in the process—also across wide taxonomic boundaries.

The bottom line is that bacteria freely and rapidly distribute hereditary material among themselves. Add to that the ease with which people travel around the world, carrying bacteria with them that might otherwise remain localized, and we have a global melting pot for bacterial gene swapping—and a recipe for disaster.

Biologists once believed that drug resistance was caused primarily by new mutations within the genetic material of the microbe—spontaneous structural changes or "errors" that made the microbe suddenly resistant. Today scientists realize that, after four billion years of making errors, most of the drug-resistant genes are out there somewhere. The problem with drug resistance is not the emergence of new genes in old germs but the teaming up of old genes with new hosts. Many of these new teams are forming deadly combinations. And the rate at which microorganisms can "mutate" is alarming. Says David Morens, medical epidemiologist at the National Institute of Allergy and Infectious Diseases (NIAID), a division of the U.S. National Institutes of Health (NIH): "When an enterovirus like polio goes through the human gastrointestinal tract in three days, its genome mutates about two percent. That level of mutation . . . has taken the human species eight million years to accomplish. So who's going to adapt to whom?"

The situation is greatly compounded by extreme overuse of antibiotics. Fifty to 60 percent of all outpatient prescriptions for antibiotics are inappropriate. David Welch, associate professor of pediatrics at the University of Oklahoma Health Services Center, says, "The effects of antibiotics, once the wonder drugs that all but wiped out killers such as tuberculosis and surgical infection, are being eroded dangerously by misuse and overprescription." It is ironic that the solution to the problem of infectious disease has become the cause.

Survival of the fittest. "Bacteria develop resistance to antibiotics for the same Darwinian reason that gazelles evolved speed in response to lions," says Sharon Begley in "The End of Antibiotics" (*Newsweek*, March 28, 1994). In a population of gazelles, slower-footed members were more easily caught, killed, and eaten. The fleetest-footed members survived in greater numbers to an age where they could reproduce. Ultimately, the slower-moving gazelles were eliminated from the population. Evolutionists would say that there was "selective pressure" created by hungry lions, leading to a reproductive advantage for the fleet-footed gazelles. The dynamics that lead to change in this way were first recognized by Darwin and are known as *natural selection* or *survival of the fittest.*

Bacteria are subject to the same dynamics as gazelles. All living things are. Within a colony of, say, *S. aureus*, most members are sensitive to penicillin. They die. Fleming observed this sensitivity on his petri dish in 1928. Most doctors experienced it when they treated soldiers and civilians with penicillin during and after World War II. The bacteria were, for the most part, penicillin-sensitive. But among the *S. aureus* population nationwide or worldwide there were some, albeit very few, that carried the gene for penicillin resistance. The widespread use of penicillin created a selective pressure, providing a reproductive advantage for the penicillin-resistant staph. In time a strain that was once very rare became all too common, and a drug that was once effective became useless. It happened to penicillin with *S. aureus* in a few short years. And it continues to happen to all antibiotics with all microbes.

The answer, of course, is not to forgo the use of drugs but just not to overprescribe them. When used judiciously, antibiotics will kill disease-causing bacteria and save lives. There is always the threat that selective pressure will cause a drug-resistant strain to raise its ugly head, but the threat increases dramatically with the increased use of antibiotics. The end justifies the means only when antibiotics are used wisely, which is not always the case. For example:

• Antibiotics are useless against viruses. Yet it is estimated that close to half the people visiting a doctor for a viral infection, such as the common cold or the flu, receive an antibiotic prescription. According to the CDC, physicians in the United States write eighteen million antibiotic prescriptions each year to treat the common cold.

• Many doctors prescribe antibiotics prophylactically, or preventively, rather than as a treatment for documented infections. Use of antibiotics in this way is rarely justified.

• Many doctors prescribe antibiotics to allay the fears and anxieties of a patient. Use of antibiotics in this way is never justified.

• In third-world nations, such as India and countries in Africa and South America, antibiotics are drastically overused. Many are dispensed by local pharmacists without prescription—and often in amounts too small to have therapeutic value but still capable of producing drug resistance. Drug-resistant strains of bacteria that emerge in these developing nations find their way to the four corners of the earth.

• Farmers overuse drugs in their livestock. Most of the meat Americans eat comes from "factory farms," assembly lines designed to raise as many animals as possible in the smallest available space, to maximize profits. With cattle or hogs or chickens crowded together over long periods, it is difficult to keep disease down. The solution: pump antibiotics into the animals. American farmers are perhaps the greatest abusers of drugs. They administer up to thirty times more antibiotics to their cattle than the average person receives. The drugs are used prophylactically and even to promote animal growth (nondiseased animals grow fatter than diseased ones). This abuse has caused dangerous drug-resistant strains of bacteria to develop. For example, humans now face a toxic strain of *E. coli*, the normally harmless resident in human and animal guts. Threatened by constant exposure to antibiotics in the feed of beef cattle, *E. coli* made use of a drug-resistant gene it had originally gotten from shigella, a nasty bug that causes dysentery. Unfortunately, it also inherited shigella's nastiness. The overuse of antibiotics created a selective pressure for the development of toxic *E. coli*. It was first detected in 1982; in 1993 it killed three children who ate hamburgers at a Jack-in-the-Box restaurant and infected at least five hundred fast-food patrons. More recently, *E coli* killed a little girl who indulged in watermelon slices at a Sizzler in Milwaukee. Scientists estimate that the bacterium hits about twenty thousand people a year. Farm-induced antibiotic resistance also includes *Campylobacter*, a bacterium that causes fever, diarrhea, and bloody stools, but is usually not fatal, and the infamous enterococcus, which often is. Each year seventy-six million Americans get sick from what they eat, and of those, five thousand die.

The Future

The obvious first step in stemming the rising tide of drug resistance is responsible use of antibiotics. It is difficult to control antibiotic distribution and use throughout the world, but agencies such as the CDC, NIH, and WHO must make greater efforts to monitor the prescribing of antibiotics and the emergence of drug-resistant strains of bacteria. The CDC—the largest institution for fighting infectious disease in the world—is encouraging local health officials to conduct regular surveys for drug resistance. WHO is funding a global computer database that doctors can use to report drug-resistant outbreaks.

But surveillance alone is not enough. The public should be educated regarding the proper and improper use of antibiotics, and doctors who are in a position to prescribe drugs should be required to take update courses on the latest developments in the field of antibiotics. Narrow-spectrum drugs should be used, where effective, rather than broad-spectrum drugs. Milder drugs should be used, where effective, rather than more potent ones. And the smallest effective dose should always be used.

There must also be a renewed commitment to antibiotic research. It is interesting that the sale of antibiotics to drugstores and hospitals in the

United States has increased steadily from $3.7 billion in 1988 to $6 billion in 1994, and more than $10 billion by the turn of the century, yet funding for antibiotic research has steadily declined. This is unfortunate, given the resourcefulness of bacteria. According to Dr. David Morens, "It takes us seventeen years to develop an antibiotic. But a bacterium can develop resistance virtually in minutes."

Space bugs. Interestingly, the National Aeronautics and Space Administration (NASA) has noticed that, under certain conditions, bacteria in the zero- or microgravity of space will produce antibiotics at a faster rate than earthbound bugs—as much as 200 percent faster. Why? Researchers believe that bacteria produce antibiotics in response to stress, and the reduced gravity of space somehow creates greater stress. On April 4, 2002, space shuttle *Atlantis* carried an experiment to the International Space Station (it returned June 19 on the *Endeavor*) to study the effects of microgravity on antibiotic production in bacteria—specifically, actinomycin D. At this writing, data from this experiment are being analyzed.

Frogs and sharks. Other avenues of prevention and treatment must also be explored. A promising line of research involves animals much higher on the evolutionary ladder than the bacteria and fungi, which have provided us with most of our antibiotics. Michael Zasloff, a researcher and former professor of medicine and genetics at the University of Pennsylvania, has discovered substances with powerful antibiotic properties in such diverse creatures as frogs and sharks. In frogs it is a milky fluid that oozes from the skin and is called *magainin*. In dogfish sharks the substance is called *squalamine*. A closer look at nature may provide us with thousands, or even millions, of chemicals with which to do battle against infectious disease. Remember, one of the first effective agents against infectious disease came from a bug in a bog in southern New Jersey.

Phages. Perhaps the most promising line of research involves organisms a bit *lower* on the evolutionary ladder than bacteria and fungi: bacteriophages. As mentioned earlier, they are viruses that infect and kill bacteria. Their therapeutic value was first recognized in 1917 by a French bacteriologist, Felix d'Hérelle, who noticed that agents thought to be viruses were killing dysentery bacteria in the bloody stools of World War II soldiers. Bacteriophage therapy was used with some success in the early 1900s in the United States but was abandoned with the advent of antibiotics. Russian scientists have used phages to fight bacterial disease for decades—mostly against *enterococcus* and other enteric and skin pathogens—and with the appearance of drug-resistant and multidrug-resistant bacteria, it is making a comeback elsewhere. One researcher has used phages to treat a seafood-related illness caused by the bacterium *Vibrio vulnificans*, which, in full-blown infection, has a 50 percent mortality rate. Experiments on mice have proven very effective. Michael H. Walter of the University of Northern Iowa has worked with phages that infect *Bacillus cereus*, a cousin of the anthrax bug. He hopes to develop phages that can be used to treat infections of anthrax, a germ that has gained recent notoriety as a weapon of bioterror. (See Chapter 11, "Bioterrorism," for more on anthrax.) Carl Merril of the NIH and Richard Carlton of Exponential Biotherapies, Inc., have developed a bacteriophage to fight antibiotic-resistant strains of enterococci, the scourge of hospitals and nursing homes. One particular phage defended mice against a vancomycin-resistant strain. "At the right dose, we get 100% survival," Carlton told *Science News*.

Dr. Vincent Fischetti, working at the Rockefeller University in New York City, has been able to purify an enzyme produced by phages to kill their host bacteria. According to Dr. Fischetti, "As little as 10 ng [.000000001 gram] of enzyme is sufficient to destroy 10 million streptococci within seconds in vitro. When small amounts of enzyme were added to the oral cavity of mice that had been intentionally colonized with group A streptococci, the enzyme destroyed all the organism being carried by the mice. We thus have developed a non-antibiotic method to control bacteria that normally cause infection."

A Baltimore biotechnology company, Intralytix, is developing a mix of salmonella-killing phages that can be sprayed on poultry in processing plants as a "disinfectant." It is also working on a phage-coated dressing, "PhageBioderm," that would be placed over wounds or burns to prevent bacterial infection. Keep in mind that most people who die of burns do so within two days—of bacterial infections.

Phages have advantages over antibiotics. They are like smart bombs, specific for only a few strains of bacteria; they usually work in a single dose, since they multiply within their host; and although a bacterium can adapt and develop resistance to a phage, the phage can adapt with it—in fact it adapts better.

Bubbles. Frogs, sharks, and phages aside, there are microbubbles. Or more correctly, *nanobubbles*. James Baker, professor of nanotechnology and medicine at the University of Michigan, and head of NanoBio, a biotech firm in Ann Arbor, has produced an emulsion of soybean in water. Think salad dressing, in which tiny bubbles of oil are suspended in vinegar. Only Baker's bubbles are super tiny, measuring one nanometer (10^{-9} meter) across, or one hundred thousand times narrower than a human hair. The bubbles store energy in their surface tension (the smaller the bubble, the greater the energy), and when they come in contact with the fatty component of bacterial membranes or viral coats, the bubbles coalesce and release their energy in nanoexplosions that tear apart the microorganism. Kind of like a nanotorpedo. Importantly, the bubbles do not harm human cells, except for red blood cells and sperm cells, because of their particular fragility.

The uses of the soy emulsion are nearly limitless. Spray it on or mix it in foods as a preservative; rub it on the skin as a cream to fight acne, athlete's foot, or other skin infections; gargle with or spray it in the nose and mouth to prevent bad breath, tooth decay, the flu, common colds, etc. Since sperm cells are vulnerable, it could be used as a contraceptive and at the same time a prophylaxis against STDs such as HIV or herpes. It has even shown to be effective against the extremely hardy and physically resistant spore stage of certain bacteria, such as the bioweapon anthrax. In controlled experiments with mice, it protected against cutaneous anthrax. For this reason, the U.S. military's Defense Advanced Research Projects Agency (DARPA) is supporting nanoemulsion research and development. It gives new meaning to the phrase, "I hate to burst your bubble."

Pathogens are a formidable enemy. They are highly adaptive and resourceful. They are the ultimate survivors. The road to defeating them will be long and tortuous and will not be journeyed without innovative, daring approaches and a superhuman commitment in both money and manpower.

4

The White Death

The common fallacy of consumptive persons, who feel not themselves dying, and therefore still hope to live.

—Sir Thomas Browne

Tuberculosis (TB) is not a new disease; it dates back at least seven thousand years, to the skeletal remains of a man whose spine had been eaten away by the disease. It may have comprised the first pestilence. It is referred to in the Bible. It was the "plague of the pharaohs." Over the last two centuries it has killed an estimated two billion people and has disfigured, crippled, and blinded countless billions more. During the late nineteenth century it killed more people in the United States than any other disease. Over the course of its gruesome history it is difficult to imagine the number of people who have suffered and died from tuberculosis.

In ancient India no Brahman was permitted to marry into a family where tuberculosis existed. In New England in the eighteenth and nineteenth centuries graves of tuberculosis victims were dug up months or even years after burial and mutilated in the hope of preventing the dead from reaching out and sucking the life force from the living. Tuberculosis has been called the *white plague*, or *white death*, killing far more people than any other pestilence. It presently infects one out of every three people in the world, or about two billion, and kills three million of those each year. Eight million new cases are reported annually. In the United States, ten to fifteen million people are infected with the tubercle bacillus, and thousands die each year. Worldwide, it remains the largest cause of death from a single pathogen.

Contrary to popular belief, Columbus did not bring tuberculosis to the New World as he did smallpox, measles, mumps, influenza, cholera, malaria, typhoid, typhus, diphtheria, and scarlet fever. An examination of the mummified remains of a Peruvian woman who lived five hundred years before Columbus set sail revealed the presence of DNA that is identical to that of the germ that causes TB. How the disease got to the Americas from Europe and Asia, and where it originated, remains a mystery.

Captain of the Men of Death

Although tuberculosis is caused by a single species of microorganism, the course of its infection is varied. (There are a number of other species that may cause a similar illness, but infection by these is rare today, except among HIV-positive or immunocompromised individuals.) The tubercle bacillus spares no part of the human body. Without treatment it is a brutal destroyer. It most commonly infects the lungs, slowly eating away the tissue, forming abscesses that continually discharge a cheesy, foul-smelling pus. The lung infection can work its way through the body wall to the surface of the chest, where it will form large ulcerations that ooze pus rich with tuberculosis germs. Over years the lungs are destroyed and the patient wastes away, becoming pale and weak and emaciated, coughing up blood, unable to breathe. A common name for the disease, *consumption*, derives from this tragic condition. Death may come ultimately—and mercifully—from lung destruction or the rupture of a major pulmonary artery, in which case the victim dies quickly from blood loss or by drowning in his or her own blood. Adolf Hitler's father died from such a hemorrhage.

As a result of swallowing one's own contaminated sputum, the tuberculosis germs may spill into the digestive tract, where they can cause painful ulcerations of the throat, making it difficult to speak or swallow. The infection can work its way down the digestive tube, infecting the stomach and bowels—where it is potentially fatal—causing bloody vomiting, bloody diarrhea, and acute pain. If it spills into the bloodstream, where it is invariably fatal without treatment (called *miliary* tuberculosis), no organ or tissue is exempt. American poet Walt Whitman died of complications from miliary tuberculosis. According to the *New York Times* (March 28, 1892), in addition to deterioration of his lungs and other organs, the poet's heart "was surrounded by a large number of small abscesses and about two and a half quarts of water."

Miliary TB can infect the urinary tract, causing extremely painful inflammation. In cases of urinary bladder infections, surgeons in the early part of the twentieth century would reconnect the tube leading from the kidneys directly to the body surface, bypassing the bladder, to relieve the unbearable pain upon urination. If the infection reached the kidneys, which it often did in cases of urinary tract infection, death would usually result from kidney failure.

It is a short trip from the urinary to the genital tract. Women are especially susceptible to this mode of infection. Without treatment the disease infiltrates their ovaries and fallopian tubes, mutilating the tissue in an ugly mass of pus, inflammation, and eventual scarring, depriving the survivors of the joys of motherhood forever.

The disease could cause fatal infection of the liver, brain, and meninges—membranes surrounding the brain and spinal cord. It could eat holes in every bone in the body, causing crippling hip, elbow, shoulder, and leg conditions. It could snap the spine, leading to the characteristic hunchback appearance of many TB sufferers. It could redden and harden the skin around the face and mouth, leading to a wolflike appearance called *lupus vulgaris*; or it could eat away the nose, ears, and eyes. In *The Forgotten Plague*, Dr. Frank Ryan describes the condition of one such victim:

> *Her face had suffered thirty years of destructive ulceration, leading to grotesque deformity. Her nose had been eaten away by degrees until there was nothing there except two gibbous caverns. Her left eye had been destroyed. Freida now looked out upon the world from a monstrously scarred mask, cratered with festering sores that teemed with tuberculosis germs. Even the comfort of*

plastic surgery had been denied to her since every graft that had been attempted had itself become infected and ultimately destroyed by invading germs.

Such is the nightmare of tuberculosis, "the captain of all these men of death," as English writer and preacher John Bunyan called consumption.

A Natural-Born Killer

The captain is a microbe called *Mycobacterium tuberculosis*. It is a rather small, rod-shaped bacterium that measures in at barely $\frac{1}{10,000}$ of an inch (.000003 meter) in length, with a thickness that makes a human hair look like a tree trunk. It doesn't swim around at all and breathes oxygen. It has a very waxy cell wall that gives it particular staining properties, called acid fast, and makes it resistant to destruction by drying and by chemical agents (direct sunlight, however, will destroy it). Consequently, tuberculosis germs that are coughed out into the air can remain alive and viable for weeks or months—much longer than most other bacteria. On the other hand, *M. tuberculosis* does not form endospores, the extremely durable resting stage of certain bacteria, such as *B. anthracis*, which is one reason why anthrax is considered a bioterrorist weapon of choice. Endospores can survive for years without food or water.

M. tuberculosis was first identified as the causative agent of the white death by Robert Koch in 1882. It was a momentous discovery. At the time, tuberculosis killed one in seven human beings and was more feared than cholera or the bubonic plague. Koch announced his discovery at a meeting of the Physiological Society in Berlin on March 24. Paul Ehrlich, the discoverer of salvarsan for syphilis, attended the meeting and later remarked: "I hold that evening to be the most important experience of my scientific life."

The identification of *M. tuberculosis* was no mean accomplishment. Researchers had been working at it for the better part of a century. Its small size and difficult staining characteristics were compounded by the fact that it grew extremely slowly. While some bacteria, such as the gut dweller *E. coli*, can multiply every twenty minutes, *M. tuberculosis* multiplies every eighteen to twenty-four hours. It can take up to eight weeks for dry, pale yellow colonies to become visible on solid medium.

The slow growth rate of *M. tuberculosis* characterizes the typical progression of the disease. It is a seductively slow killer. In *Nicholas Nickleby*, Charles Dickens describes it as a "gradual, quiet, and solemn" killer that wastes and withers away the body. Unlike influenza, which killed by conservative estimates more than twenty million people during the winter of 1918–19, or epidemics of smallpox and bubonic plague, which run their course in weeks or months, or the hemorrhagic diseases like Ebola and Marburg, or aggressive, flesh-eating strep A, which kill within days or even hours, tuberculosis takes years—often many years—to take its toll. Thousands of years of evolution have turned it into a clever parasite; it feasts at the dinner table for a long while before killing off its meal ticket.

Also, it is not as certain a killer as many other infectious diseases. Ninety percent of those who are infected with the most virulent strain of Ebola virus die of it; they bleed to death from every opening in their body. And virtually all of those who contract rabies succumb to it. Not so with tuberculosis. About one in ten who become infected actually becomes ill with the disease—or gets *active TB*. (Of those, about half will die within five years without treatment.) The remaining nine out of ten infected people, especially those without depressed immune systems, are able to fight the disease and wall off the infection. These people have *inactive TB*. The walled-off nodule is called a *tubercle*, from its resemblance to a tuber, and gives the disease its name. However, the tubercle bacilli have the lethal potential to break through the wall and reactivate, often many years later— and with a vengeance.

The incidence of active TB increases dramatically during times of war, famine, or social/economic depression. Its tragic association with AIDS will be addressed at the end of the chapter.

An Equal-Opportunity Destroyer

M. tuberculosis is a close cousin of the germ that causes leprosy, *M. leprae*, and of several nonpathogenic microbes that dwell in the soil. It is most commonly transmitted from person to person by droplet infection—when someone with active TB coughs, sneezes, or speaks and sprays into the air droplets laden with tuberculosis germs. (It is important to note that only a person with active TB is infectious.) The disease is not as contagious as the common cold or the flu, which are also spread by droplet infection, and is not generally spread by touching articles that have been handled by actively infected people.

But its communicability should never be underestimated. In the spring of 1994, four passengers were infected by a woman with active TB during an eight-and-a-half-hour United Airlines flight from Chicago to Honolulu. It was the first documented case of tuberculosis transmission from one person to another on a commercial airline and serves as a painful reminder that tuberculosis is indeed a contagious disease.

Milk is also a source of human infection, especially among children, causing bone, intestinal, and miliary tuberculosis and tuberculosis in the lymph nodes in the neck (called *scrofula*), which erupts on the surface of the skin as pus-filled sores.* However, with the testing of cows for infection and the widespread practice of milk pasteurization, tuberculosis from contaminated milk is rare. It accounts for less than 1 percent of tuberculosis cases in the United States.

More than any other disease, tuberculosis has disrupted the fabric of society. It has been a disease of the rich as well as the poor, the privileged as well as the deprived, the haves as well as the have-nots. It has been the scourge of developed nations as well as third-world countries. Its reign of terror throughout history, and the typically protracted manner in which it claims its victims, have imbued tuberculosis with a kind of mystical, if morbid, fascination—inspiring great literature and music. Thomas Mann's Nobel Prize–winning novel, *The Magic Mountain*, is set in a tuberculosis sanatorium in the Swiss Alps. Little Blossom in Dickens's *David Copperfield* dies of consumption, as does Mimi in Puccini's opera *La Bohème*. Verdi's opera *La Traviata* is centered around a consumptive beauty, Violetta, a character based on Marguerite Gauthier, the heroine in Alexandre Dumas's *La Dame aux Camélias*.

Tuberculosis has infected and claimed the lives of many renowned real-life personalities as well. In particular it has impacted on the arts, killing a staggering number of the world's greatest writers and composers at the height of their creative genius. Table 2 is a short "Who's Who" of famous—and infamous—tuberculosis victims (in chronological order by birth).

---

*Milk-borne TB is actually caused by *M. bovis*, a close relative of *M. tuberculosis*. It is believed that *M. bovis* evolved first and became parasitic in animals that breathed it in from the air or ingested it from the soil as they grazed. Humans picked it up by drinking infected milk or eating infected meat. It eventually mutated to *M. tuberculosis*, the more common human pathogen.

Table 2 *Famous People Who Suffered from Tuberculosis*

Name	Occupation	Birth–Death
King Tutankhamen* (and many other pharaohs)	Egyptian pharaoh	ca. 1358–1340 B.C.
Cardinal Richelieu*	French statesman	1585–1642
Jean Molière*	French playwright	1622–1673
Baruch Spinoza*	Dutch philosopher	1632–1677
François Voltaire	French writer/philosopher	1749–1832
Johann Goethe	German writer/scientist	1749–1832
Johann Schiller*	German writer/historian	1759–1805
Sir Walter Scott*	Scottish novelist/poet	1771–1832
Niccolò Paganini	Italian violin virtuoso	1782–1840
Simón Bolívar*	Venezuelan revolutionary leader	1783–1830
John Keats*	English poet	1795–1821
Ralph Waldo Emerson	American essayist/poet	1803–1882
Elizabeth Barrett Browning*	English poet	1806–1861
Edgar Allan Poe*	American story writer/poet	1809–1849
Frédéric Chopin*	Polish composer/pianist	1810–1849
Emily Brontë*	English novelist/poet	1818–1848
Walt Whitman*	American poet	1819–1892
Fyodor Dostoyevsky	Russian novelist	1821–1881
Paul Gauguin	French painter	1848–1903
Robert Louis Stevenson*	Scottish writer	1850–1894
Anton Chekhov*	Russian writer	1860–1904
Franz Kafka	Czech novelist	1883–1924
Eleanor Roosevelt*	American humanitarian/first lady	1884–1962
D. H. Lawrence*	English writer	1885–1930
Eugene O'Neill*	American playwright	1888–1953
Adolf Hitler	German dictator	1889–1945
George Orwell*	English novelist/essayist	1903–1950
Vivien Leigh*	English actress	1913–1967
Nelson Mandela	African nationalist leader	1918–

*Died of tuberculosis

Winning the Battle

Twenty-four hundred years ago the Greek physician Hippocrates—who considered tuberculosis the deadliest of all diseases—treated consumptives with a soothing diet of honey, barley gruel, and wine. Later cultures treated tubercular patients less kindly, viewing the disease as a form of demonic possession and resorting to more drastic measures to exorcise the evil spirits. In the extreme, treatments approached the comical. They included attaching a dead fish to the sufferer's chest or having the sufferer suckle milk from a human breast.

In 1908 a vaccine against tuberculosis was developed.

An Ounce of Prevention

The vaccine was developed by two French scientists, Albert Calmette and Camille Guérin, using a weakened, avirulent strain of the germ that causes tuberculosis in cattle, *M. bovis* (footnoted earlier). It is known as the Bacillus Calmette-Guérin (BCG) vaccine and is the most widely used vaccine in the world. It remains the only vaccine currently available against tuberculosis, but nobody is certain how well it works—or if it does at all.

No fewer than eighteen large-scale, carefully controlled studies of BCG immunization have been carried out in the United States and other countries, including a fifteen-year study by the World Health Organization (WHO). In some trials the vaccine has been shown to protect 80 percent of those vaccinated, while in others it has provided no protection at all.

These widely disparate results are indeed baffling and have prompted different countries to adopt different policies concerning the vaccine's use. It is most widely used in developing nations, where tuberculosis is prevalent and the risk of infection high. It is also used, though more selectively, in Great Britain, Europe, and most other developed nations, especially among children in families where members have active tuberculosis, and among doctors, nurses, and health care workers who come in contact with tuberculosis sufferers. It is not used, or recommended for use, in one country in the world—the United States.

There are reasons for this aside from the conflicting reports on its efficacy. First of all, a person who receives the BCG vaccine will test positive with the tuberculin skin test. This test (discussed later in the chapter) is used by health organizations as a powerful tool for detecting infection at an early stage and for assessing the spread of the disease. BCG renders this test useless. Second, it cannot be given to people who are HIV-positive. Though the BCG bacillus is harmless to a person with an intact immune system, it can cause TB in one whose immune system has been compromised.

Also, the BCG vaccine—where it has been shown to work—can protect only people who are uninfected, not infected but inactive. And it does not protect them from infection but only from the more serious or life-threatening complications of the disease. Health officials argue that the vaccine lowers such risk in children more than in adults. (BCG is now being given to more than 80 percent of the world's children.)

Last, American epidemiologists note that the protection conferred by BCG is often short-lived and provides no convincing argument that its use has any impact on the total control of tuberculosis in any country.

But the disease is rising at an alarming rate worldwide. The discouraging statistics have caused federal health officials in the United States to rethink their position on the use of BCG. A serious effort is being made to determine if BCG might be more effective than its critics admit. In the meantime, research is being done to find out why some strains of the BCG germ seem to work while others do not and to develop an entirely new antituberculosis vaccine. Microbiologist Marcus Horowitz and his colleagues at the UCLA School of Medicine have done testing of a vaccine composed not of the entire TB germ but of key proteins that make it up. It is a relatively new concept of vaccination: target specific immunologically active sites rather than the whole microbe—a biological smart bomb. Horowitz has shown the "protein vaccine" to be effective in immunizing laboratory animals against TB. Human testing is the next step.

When the medical establishment cannot adequately protect people from disease, the next best thing is to treat the disease effectively, limiting its spread and minimizing the pain, suffering, debilitation, and death that it would normally cause. Tuberculosis has an interesting history in this regard.

A Breath of Fresh Air

A serious approach to treating tuberculosis began in the mid-1800s. An English doctor, George Bodington, observed that people who lived in rural areas were much less susceptible to TB than people who lived in major cities. He attributed this statistic to the fact that country air was cleaner and fresher than city air. A German doctor, Hermann Brehmer, heard of Bodington's fresh-air theory and was impressed. In 1859, at Görbersdorf in the Silesian Mountains, he built a small sanatorium for tuberculosis victims. It was the first of its kind. To the prescription of fresh air he added rest, an exercise regimen, a healthful diet—and an occasional cocktail or two. The concept that consumption could be cured by total rest in the open air caught on, and throughout the latter part of the 1800s sanatoriums sprang up all across Europe, where tuberculosis was responsible for one in

every four deaths. They were, in effect, health spas for the tubercular. Davos, in the Swiss Alps, was recognized as a choice location for inhaling "pure air" and became a mecca for tuberculosis patients. Many prominent men and women, including Robert Louis Stevenson and the wife of Sir Arthur Conan Doyle, flocked to the sanatoriums there.

In the United States the first sanatorium was opened by Dr. Edward Livingston Trudeau in the Adirondack Mountains of New York. It was located on the shores of idyllic Flower Lake, near the Saranac and St. Regis chains of lakes. Dr. Trudeau, a tuberculosis victim himself, had gone to the Saranac Lake region in 1873, prepared to die. Surprisingly, he recovered. Attributing his good fortune to the salubrious effects of the clean, brisk Adirondack air, he set up a sanatorium, which was opened to the public in 1884. (He also founded the first tuberculosis research facility in the United States, in 1894.) As with the sanatoriums at Davos, the Trudeau Sanatorium attracted a host of people, including again Robert Louis Stevenson, Hall of Fame baseball pitcher "Christy" Mathewson, and Albert Einstein, who was not himself a tuberculosis sufferer. As had happened in Europe, the success of Trudeau's sanatorium prompted the construction of many others across America. Every county in every state seemed to have one. By the turn of the century the sanatorium had become an established institution in both American and European society. Some were private and exclusive, others public and modest. Some were relaxed in their program— little more than vacations with a medical stamp of approval—while others ran a spartan operation. In *Saranac: America's Magic Mountain*, Robert Taylor quotes from a Davos sanatorium guidebook of 1880: "Consumption has always been too timorously, too leniently, too indulgently dealt with. Davos demands qualities the very opposite of resigned sentimentalism. . . . Here is no place for weak and despairing resignation; here you are not pusillanimously helped to die, but are required to enter into a hard struggle for life."

Likewise, the Trudeau Sanatorium implemented an active, demanding program of self-help for its patients. For their efforts they are to be commended, but did the sanatoriums really work? Did they really cure people of tuberculosis? Did they lower the death rate, mitigate the suffering? To all a qualified yes. Undoubtedly fresh air, rest, healthful food, and reduc-

tion of stress helped those with TB to fight off the infection. Rest and proper nutrition led to a healthier constitution, which in turn led to a healthier immune system. (Poor health and nutrition, in fact, contribute to the growing threat of tuberculosis today.) At the Trudeau, 12,500 patients were cared for during its seventy years of operation. When it closed its doors in 1954, 5,000 of those patients were still alive. Most impressive, considering how many may have died of complications associated with old age or other non-TB-related causes during that considerable span of time.

The sanatoriums reduced spread of the disease as well. Most patients remained at a sanatorium for at least a year, some for most of their adult life. It served as an effective quarantine, removing those with active and contagious tuberculosis from the mainstream population.

Today the sanatoriums are gone—footnotes to medical history and colorful reminders of an era that once was. They closed their doors, very simply, because they ran out of customers. The Trudeau treated only sixty patients in its closing year and ran a deficit of ninety thousand dollars. In the United States, by the mid-1950s, tuberculosis took only 6 percent of the lives that it had in 1900. The reason for this dramatic decline? Antibiotics.

Chemical Warfare

Before the advent of antibiotics the outlook for many tuberculosis sufferers was rather bleak, sanatoriums notwithstanding. Surgery was one option. A lung, an eye, a major portion of one's rib cage were often removed in cases where infection was aggressive and tissue destruction extensive. For pulmonary tuberculosis, methods were devised to rest the infected lung or lungs by reducing a person's ability to take a deep breath. In one approach, artificial pneumothorax, a long, hollow needle was inserted between the ribs and air pumped into the chest cavity to create pressure from outside the lung, keeping it partially deflated. In the extreme the lung could be completely collapsed, affording it a better opportunity to heal. In place of air, objects such as rubber balls or Ping-Pong balls were sometimes placed inside the chest cavity—which was surgically opened and then closed—to provide a physical barrier to breathing. In the most severe cases, ribs were removed—as many as eight or nine—in a highly invasive and disfiguring operation to keep the lung permanently collapsed.

In another method nerves leading to the diaphragm, a muscle that controls breathing, would be crushed or severed to impair their function and limit breathing capacity.

These procedures worked to a very limited degree. If the body did not successfully combat the infection, walling it off in a tubercle, the patient was in serious trouble.

Extremely helpful in the early detection of TB, both during the sanatorium days and today, is the tuberculin skin test, also known as the Mantoux test. Tuberculin is a protein derivative of the tuberculosis bacterium. It was discovered by Robert Koch in 1890. In the tuberculin test a very small amount of the protein is introduced under the skin. The body of a person who has been infected with tuberculosis will be sensitive to the protein, and the skin around the site of injection will become red and swollen within forty-eight to seventy-two hours. In young children a positive tuberculin test often means active tuberculosis. However, in older people it might indicate a sensitivity resulting from a previous infection that has since become inactive. As mentioned earlier, a person who has received a tuberculosis vaccine will also test positive. False positives may also result from cross-reactions with other substances that stimulate the immune system or from contaminated tuberculin. In all cases of positive tuberculin skin tests, a chest x-ray is indicated to determine if there has been an actual infection and, if so, its status and the extent of damage it has caused.

Although tuberculin remains an invaluable diagnostic tool, its discovery was accompanied by misfortune. In tuberculin Koch thought he had found a cure for the dreaded White Death. He announced this to the world. Tuberculin became available worldwide and was used by doctors in large doses to treat their tubercular patients. Unfortunately, it aggravated the disease instead of curing it. Many people died as a result of Koch's tuberculin treatment. His reputation was ruined; police were needed to protect him from angry crowds. It is uncertain how he could have made such an egregious error in his evaluation of tuberculin, but the consequences proved a sad and undeserved ending to the life and career of one of the greatest figures in the history of medicine. Koch died on May 27, 1910, of a heart attack and a broken heart.

The defeat of tuberculosis would come thirty-four years later, not with tuberculin but with antibiotics. The earliest of these, penicillin and Prontosil, were not effective against TB. But by the mid-1940s three drugs were discovered that did have important antituberculosis activity: streptomycin, para-aminosalicylic acid (PAS), and Conteben. Of the three, streptomycin would achieve historical importance as the first to be used as an effective treatment. The drug was administered to a human being on November 20, 1944. The patient was a twenty-one-year-old white female with advanced pulmonary tuberculosis. Her condition was deteriorating rapidly, and there was no hope for survival. Over four and a half months she received five courses of streptomycin. The pulmonary tuberculosis was arrested, and she experienced no subsequent relapses. She became the mother of three children and lived happily ever after. It was one of the millions of miracle endings to the streptomycin story.

But at exactly the same time that streptomycin was performing its wonders, another drug, PAS, was also conquering tuberculosis. It was discovered in 1943 by a brilliant Scandinavian doctor, Jorgen Lehmann, at the Sahlgren's Hospital in Göteborg, Sweden, and was as effective against tuberculosis as streptomycin. Moreover, it was first used to treat a human consumptive on October 30, 1944, three weeks before streptomycin. The patient's name was Sigrid, and she was in a state of steady decline. The disease had eaten a large hole in her right lung; she was running a high fever, had no appetite, had severe diarrhea and abdominal pains, had blood in her sputum, and was losing weight rapidly. Her attending physician had no doubt that Sigrid would soon die.

Then treatment with PAS was begun. She was given the drug orally. By March 1945 she was strong enough to undergo a major operation to repair the hole in her lung. In time she made a full and miraculous recovery. As with streptomycin, PAS would prove over and over to be a wonder drug against the White Death. Because it was taken orally, it was particularly effective against intestinal TB.

Yet in the early years after its discovery, PAS did not share the reputation of streptomycin on the world stage. Part of the problem lay in the fact that the people involved in the discovery and clinical trials of PAS—including Lehmann—were extremely slow to publish and very guarded in their appraisal of the drug. The first paper describing the remarkable antitubercular potential of PAS did not appear until January 1946, a full two years after it had been used in the first successful animal experiments. Reports on streptomycin did not suffer this delay. Also, PAS was structurally similar to aspirin, a common over-the-counter drug. It suffered guilt by association. How could an aspirin cure the world's most dreaded disease? But it did. And it did so before any of the others.

The third of these "others" was Conteben. It was discovered by Gerhard Domagk as an extension of his Nobel Prize–winning work with the sulfa drugs. The people of Germany—and Europe in general—had suffered greatly during the war. Disease, as it always does during times of human tribulation, had exacted a heavy toll—tuberculosis in particular. "Nothing could be of greater urgency in Germany today than to find a cure for tuberculosis," Domagk wrote in his diary.

He focused the attention of his research toward that end. An ingenious chemist in his employ, Robert Behnisch, tinkered with the sulfa compounds and came up with a new family of drugs, the *thiosemicarbazones* (*TSCs*). Of the thousands of TSCs that he and others put together, one in particular was effective against tuberculosis—Conteben. It was more than effective; in animal tests it cured guinea pigs infected with fatal doses of the most virulent strains of TB.

Human testing of Conteben began in 1946. Initially there were problems with dosages, and there were side effects in some patients, but the good far outdistanced the bad. Between 1947 and 1949 in Germany, twenty thousand tubercular people were treated with Conteben, and a majority of those lives were saved.

The war prevented Conteben from gaining the international exposure that it deserved. Curiously, it was not until 1949—four years after the war ended—that Conteben caught the attention of the outside world. In the autumn of that year two American doctors traveled to Germany to investigate reports of a new synthetic substance that was curing people of the White Death. Samples of the drug were taken back to the United States, where large-scale trials were carried out. It was found to be less effective than streptomycin against blood-borne tuberculosis and tuberculosis meningitis, but more effective against tuberculosis of the throat and bowels. American drug companies manufactured the product in large quantity without any compensation to Bayer, the pharmaceutical house where Conteben was discovered.

Medically, what had happened was quite remarkable. Within a few short years, and from different corners of the world, three wonder drugs had been found that could cure public disease-enemy number one. In time, other, more effective drugs would be discovered. One of these, isoniazid or INH (also discovered by the remarkable Domagk and his research team, in 1952), was found to be ten times more effective against TB than any other drug. It was the fourth of the wonder drugs against the disease. It had very few side effects and was much simpler than the other three to put together, lowering the cost of effective treatment at the time from $3,500 per patient to less than $100. It replaced Conteben and remains one of the most commonly used agent against tuberculosis. Two other frontline drugs, rifampin and ethambutol, replaced streptomycin and PAS respectively (though streptomycin is still used to a limited extent).

According to a "Fact Sheet" issued by the National Institute of Allergy and Infectious Diseases (NIAID), standard "short course" treatment today usually combines INH and rifampin, which are given for at least six months, and pyrazinamide and ethambutol (or streptomycin), which are used only in the first two months of treatment.

The drugs of choice likely will continue to change as research uncovers increasingly effective therapies. A veritable arsenal of antituberculosis drugs are presently on the market.

Between 1945 and the mid-1980s tuberculosis declined in the United States and other developed nations. The sanatoriums became redundant and were gone by the 1960s. Health organizations such as WHO, NIH, the CDC, and the U.S. National Tuberculosis Association were confidently predicting the elimination of tuberculosis, with a worldwide campaign of tuberculin testing, x-ray diagnosis, and drug therapy.

Sadly, the prediction has not been realized. From the mid-1980s to the early 1990s, the incidence of tuberculosis went up 12 percent (and double that among children) in the United States, and much more in Europe and developing nations. War, famine, overpopulation, and poor sanitation and health care have certainly contributed to this increase. But these conditions have always existed in varying degrees. What happened that was new and unexpected was, to sound a familiar refrain, *resistance*.

Losing the War

After the discovery of streptomycin Selman Waksman became a celebrated figure. He received invitations from leaders around the world to visit their country and witness the miracle of his creation. On one of these visits to France in 1947, Waksman was introduced to two young children whose lives had been saved by streptomycin. They ran up to Waksman and kissed his hand in gratitude, and he was brought to tears. They had made what the director of the hospital called "a complete recovery"—except that one year later the boy, Michael, was dead from a relapse of the disease.

It was a pattern that was becoming depressingly familiar. Initially the drug would prove miraculously effective. The patient would seem to be cured. But ultimately the germs would rise again with an armor of resistance, and the patient would relapse and then die. Nor was resistance limited to streptomycin. Tuberculosis bacteria have become resistant to every anti-TB drug developed. Germs have an uncanny ability to adapt and survive. TB germs were found in the laboratory that were not only resistant to streptomycin, but were using it as a source of nutrition, actually preferring it to their customary food.

People with drug-resistant TB may be prescribed more than a dozen medications—often with serious side effects—for a period of up to twenty-four months, in the hope that the combination might arrest infection. In the most stubborn cases a lung may be collapsed or removed, along with ribs and sections of the lining of the chest wall. Nerves leading to the diaphragm may be crushed or air pumped into the abdominal cavity to restrict breathing, helping a diseased lung heal. These are treatments reminiscent of the pre-antibiotic days of the early twentieth century. According to Dr. Michael Iseman, chief of the TB service at the National Jewish Center in Denver, Colorado, which gets many of the nation's most severe drug-resistant cases, "We are willing to gamble on very painful and risky treatments because this is their last shot. If we can't control their disease, they die the death of consumption, slowly strangled as the TB eats away at their lungs" (*New York Times*, October 12, 1992).

The cure rate at National Jewish is astounding—about 90 percent. Nationwide, without the elaborate and very expensive treatment offered at the hospital (which can cost up to $250,000 for one patient), as many as 50 percent of those afflicted with resistant TB die a miserable death.

The statistics are alarming, and drug-resistant TB is not going away. In inner-city hospitals today one in three new cases of TB is found to be drug-resistant; but more frightening is that one in five is found to be multiple-drug-resistant (MDR). From 1993 to 1997, forty-three states and the District of Columbia reported cases of multidrug-resistant TB.

A Drug-Resistant Bug

When tuberculosis was last common in this country, drug resistance was exceedingly rare. Antibiotics and chemotherapies against TB had not yet been discovered. There was no selective advantage for drug-resistant bacteria. In general, bacteria with no drug resistance are hardier creatures—save for their drug sensitivity—and will predominate in a given population. This holds true for *M. tuberculosis*. Before anti-TB drugs came on the scene, drug-sensitive TB germs were the predominant cause of tuberculosis infection. Then streptomycin, PAS, and Conteben were discovered, followed half a dozen years later by isoniazid. This dramatically changed conditions on the playing field. Let's see how.

A person with a run-of-the-mill, non-drug-resistant form of tuberculosis is placed on streptomycin. The bacteria that are sensitive to the drug are wiped out, and the patient makes a remarkable recovery. However, within the population there may be a few bugs that have mutated a year ago or a million years ago and are resistant to streptomycin. They multiply unimpeded and cause a relapse of the disease six months or a year after the patient has been "cured."

The application of several drugs in combination proved extremely successful against drug-resistant TB germs at first. This is because TB germs that were drug-resistant were resistant to only one drug. In 1948 the British Medical Research Council conducted a study in which streptomycin and PAS were given in combination to a group of tubercular patients. It was the first attempt at combination therapy. The results were unequivocally successful. The long-term reduction of infection far exceeded that in groups that received streptomycin or PAS alone.

The explanation for the success is simple: those germs resistant to streptomycin were knocked out by PAS; those resistant to PAS were knocked out by streptomycin. Each drug "watched the back" of the other, so to speak. The drug-resistant TB problem should have been solved. But it wasn't. Drug-resistant TB remains a major problem today.

Incomplete or incorrect drug treatment is the reason. Take, for example, a patient—call him John—who is being given INH and rifampin. Each kills off the germs that are resistant to the other drug. However, INH is causing occasional nausea. John's TB seems to be gone; he has already been taking the drug for two months. He *must* be cured. So he decides to stop taking the INH.

But the TB germs resistant to rifampin have not been eliminated from his body. INH has been stopped too soon. As a result, rifampin-resistant germs multiply and cause a relapse of John's tuberculosis. INH is no longer there to knock them out.

John's doctor now adds a third drug to his treatment, let us say ethambutol. He does not know that John has stopped taking INH. Germs that are already resistant to rifampin are now exposed to ethambutol. Most of these rifampin-resistant germs are killed off by the new drug, but a few may have, through genetic mutation, acquired resistance to ethambutol; they adapt and flourish. Exposure to the drug has provided the selective advantage. The end result is a bug that is resistant not to one but two drugs.

A closer look at the population dynamics reveals that the large number of rifampin-resistant bugs caused by stopping INH prematurely has created the situation for double-drug resistance. With a large rifampin-resistant population, it is likely that a few of those are also ethambutol resistant. If treatment with INH was not cut short, rifampin-resistant bugs would never have increased in large numbers. In small numbers, it is very improbable that there would be ethambutol-resistant members in the bug population (statistically negligible).

The newly created rifampin/ethambutol-resistant germ can be spread to other individuals, where, through repetition of the same mechanism, it may become resistant to a third drug, and so on. Incomplete drug therapy has created a host of Frankenstein's monsters—bugs with multiple-drug resistance that have never existed before. In rare cases a TB germ may be resistant to nearly all the drugs that can be thrown at it. Resistance to three or four drugs is not uncommon. MDR TB is enormously more difficult and expensive to treat than single-drug-resistant or the once-common nonre-sistant TB infection.

To solve the problem of MDR TB, incomplete drug treatment must be addressed. One solution that seems to be working is *directly observed treatment (DOT)*. In this procedure, medical personnel are dispatched to hospital or home and literally watch the patient swallow his or her medicine every time it must be taken, and record the patient's progress for the duration of treatment—which is commonly six to nine months. DOT was tested by WHO in New York City and parts of Tanzania and China, where drug-resistant TB is a particular problem. The experiment was extremely successful. The cure rate was as high as 91 percent at some locations. DOT has been cited as one of the most cost-effective strategies ever devised against a major killer. By the end of 2000, 148 of 210 countries were implementing the DOT strategy, an increase of 21 countries since 1999. Where used in Asia, Africa, and Latin America, DOT has produced an average cure rate of 80 percent.

In New York City, DOT has reduced TB by 21 percent since 1992. In fact, due to a focused public health effort on the prevention and treatment of TB in the United States, there has been a steady decline of the disease over the past decade. Still, more than sixteen thousand cases were reported in the United States in 2000.

WHO estimates that implementing a DOT program worldwide for tuberculosis would cost about $360 million per year. Is it worth it?

Without a doubt, according to Dr. Iseman and most other TB experts and epidemiologists. It is cost-effective to spend whatever must be spent to prevent the disease from becoming multiple-drug-resistant. Dr. Iseman goes so far as to recommend giving TB patients up to twenty dollars a day as an incentive to take their medicines until they are cured. The cost of caring for patients with partly treated TB that has become multiple-drug-resistant is enormously greater.

Another problem that has compounded drug resistance is exceedingly slow growth rate of the germ. It can take up to three months to determine which antibiotics are effective against a particular strain of TB. Within the last several years, however, scientists have developed a technique using bioluminescence, in which TB germs are made to glow, becoming visible at a much earlier stage in their growth. This has enabled doctors to determine drug sensitivity in the bacteria in a matter of days.

In the United States, the Department of Health and Human Services, in collaboration with the CDC and various other medical organizations, has set a national goal to eliminate TB by the year 2010. Worldwide, WHO had originally set a goal that 70 percent of all infectious cases of TB be diagnosed, and 85 percent of those be successfully treated, by 2005. As of the latest WHO report (March 2002), that target will not be realized until 2013.

The Wolf and the Lamb

M. tuberculosis is an opportunist. It exploits weakness. It may lurk hidden and undetected in an individual for many years; then, suddenly, when the person's defenses are down, it will strike. These defenses—the immune system, to be exact—can be brought down in different ways: by certain therapies, such as radiation or chemotherapy; by poor health, brought on by improper nutrition, poverty, homelessness, and a lack of adequate health care; by continued reinfection, brought on by institutional living and general overcrowding; and by illness. The most frightening and potentially devastating illness with regard to TB is a relatively new disease, one that literally wipes out a person's immune system: AIDS. It has created a scenario that is indeed chilling.

Laurie Garrett, in *The Coming Plague*, says, "On average, infected people had a 10 percent chance of developing active [tuberculosis] sometime during their lives, and a 1 percent chance of coming down with a lethal TB illness." Thus, of the approximately 2 billion people infected with the germ, 200 million should get the disease and 20 million should die of it.

Not so. The prevalence of AIDS has turned these numbers around. Many more will become ill, and many more will die. AIDS destroys those cells in the body that combat the tuberculosis infection and wall it off. Of the 90 percent of those infected who do not normally develop active TB, most who have AIDS or are even HIV-positive do. Also, AIDS changes the very nature of the beast. *M. tuberculosis* is generally a slow, if methodical, killer. In AIDS patients it kills with the speed of an acute bacterial infection. Also, AIDS has turned a form of tuberculosis normally found only in birds into a lethal human infection—*Mycobacterium avium* complex, or MAC.

To compound the problem, studies have shown that not only does infection with HIV activate latent TB, but TB activates HIV, turning a non-symptomatic HIV-positive infection into full-blown AIDS within a few months. To quote Dr. Frank Ryan, "The twin plagues of AIDS and tuberculosis [have] come together in a synergy of terror never seen before in medical history."

The bleakest outlook exists in the developing nations. In Southeast Asia close to six million people are estimated to be HIV-positive. India alone numbers nearly two million. Many of these people are also infected with tuberculosis.

Africa is in the greatest danger of all. Presently more than two hundred million Africans, largely sub-Saharan, are infected with inactive tuberculosis. Twenty-five million are HIV-positive. The dire statistics have prompted one expert at WHO to state, with despair, "Africa is lost."

If Africa is lost, then we are all lost, for no area of the world stands alone. The spread of disease is a global phenomenon. As a human race, we are facing the greatest public health disaster in recorded history.

5

New Kids on the Block

It's no longer a question of staying healthy. It's a question of finding a sickness you like.

—JACKIE MASON

MANY INFECTIOUS DISEASES are ancient. Tuberculosis dates back seven millennia or more, to the dawn of civilization. Abscesses caused by bacteria and viruses have been found in the earliest human ancestors, dating back three million years. They have been found in birds, dating back to the age of the dinosaurs. They have been found in the earliest and simplest forms of animal and plant life, dating back more than two billion years. In fact bacteria have been found inside other bacteria, the earliest forms of life, dating back close to four billion years. Disease by infection—as noted in Chapter 1, "The Origin of Disease"—apparently is nearly as old as life itself.

But not all infectious diseases are old. Microbes are constantly changing, adapting to new situations, finding new places to live, new ways to survive. In the process once-harmless strains may turn deadly, or deadly strains may turn from other hosts to humans. AIDS is the most outstanding example. It was unheard of before 1980. Ebola, a horrible hemorrhagic disease, was unheard of before 1976. There are a number of such diseases, both bacterial and viral that, like AIDS and Ebola, are twentieth-century phenomena. They are the new kids on the block—and some of them are among the quickest and most violent killers the world has ever known. This chapter will look at some bacterial diseases that have evolved or become significant within the last few decades and have made headline news within the last several years. The viral diseases, such as Ebola and Marburg, will be discussed in Chapter 7, "Emerging Viruses"—as well as mad cow disease, which is neither viral nor bacterial but caused by a frightening new agent that is simpler than the simplest virus and more durable than an anthrax spore. AIDS has a chapter all of its own.

Lyme Disease: Getting Ticked Off

Certain diseases are spread to humans by insects or insectlike animals called *arthropods*—organisms that crawl with jointed legs and crunch when you step on them. A mosquito transmits the deadly malaria; a fly transmits sleeping sickness; a flea transmits bubonic plague; a louse transmits typhus; a tick transmits Rocky Mountain spotted fever. The list goes on. More than two hundred diseases are transmitted to humans by arthropods, which are affectionately known as "pests." Pest-borne diseases have caused many of our most serious pandemics. Through pest control, improved sanitation and hygiene, and antibiotics, most pest-borne diseases have been brought under control in the developed nations of the world. One that has not is Lyme disease. In the United States it is the first pest-borne epidemic of the post–World War II era. Between 1982 and 2000, more than 150,000 cases were reported to the CDC nationwide, but due to misdiagnosis it is believed that the actual number of cases is much greater. And each year the number increases. The CDC considers Lyme disease the most significant tick-borne disease in the United States. Eight out of every hundred thousand Americans are affected annually. In Europe it is even more widespread.

History

Lyme disease first appeared in Lyme, Connecticut, in October 1975. Several people complained to their doctor of feeling fatigued, having pain in their joints, and noticing an unusual rash on their body. Also, several children were reported to have come down with juvenile rheumatoid arthritis (JRA). Dr. Allen C. Steere, a rheumatologist at the Yale University Medical School, was dispatched to Lyme to investigate. He found thirty-nine reported cases of JRA. Something was wrong. In a community the size of Lyme, one case of JRA would be a lot. It is not a communicable disease.

Dr. Steere proceeded to interview the victims of the disease. In all cases symptoms first developed during the summer months, when people would be outdoors. Lyme was also a rural town, with many heavily wooded areas. Dr. Steere concluded that the disease was transmitted by some type of arthropod—most likely a flea, tick, mosquito, or louse. He gave it the name *Lyme disease*, or *Lyme arthritis*, after the town in which it was first observed.

Dr. Steere then studied the blood of the Lyme disease victims in an attempt to identify the causative agent, which he suspected to be a virus. He was not successful. However, he was able to identify the arthropod vector, or carrier. The culprit was an orange-brown tick called *Ixodes*. Nine of his patients had remembered being bitten by a tick that summer. One had removed it and given it to him for examination. About half a dozen species of *Ixodes* carry Lyme disease.

In 1981 Willy Burgdorfer, an international authority on tick-borne diseases, was called in. He examined the contents of the digestive tract of *Ixodes* using a technique called dark-field microscopy and found it to be teeming with a slender corkscrew-shaped microbe. The causative agent was not a virus but a bacterium—a spirochete—the same type of organism that causes syphilis. The Lyme disease spirochete was small and delicate, difficult to see and difficult to grow. It was a member of the genus *Borrelia* but unlike any *Borrelia* previously observed. In 1984, in honor of its discoverer, it was given the name *Borrelia burgdorferi*. Today, more than eighty different strains of *B. burgdorferi* have been identified worldwide.

A Tick's Life

Unlike fleas, lice, mosquitoes, flies, ants, bees, and wasps, ticks are not insects; they are arachnids. In other words, they belong to the same group as spiders, scorpions, and mites. As adults, ticks have eight legs, whereas insects have six.

Ticks are ectoparasites; they live *on* rather than *in* their host, which is usually a warm-blooded animal—a bird or mammal. They feed by embedding their mouthparts in the animal's skin and sucking its blood, like a vampire. They can't fly, and they are weak crawlers. Their life cycle consists of three stages: child (larva), adolescent (nymph), and adult.

In the case of *Ixodes* the cycle takes about two years to complete. Sean Mactire, in *Lyme Disease and Other Pest-Borne Illnesses*, describes it:

> *After the female has taken a meal of blood, it drops off to the ground and . . . proceeds to lay eggs. . . . Larvae with three pairs of legs hatch from the eggs. After a resting period, the larvae climb up to the tips of blades of grass or other plants, and wait for a host to feed on. . . . When they succeed in finding a suitable host . . . they embed their mouthparts in the skin. They remain attached for three to four days while taking a blood meal, and then drop off to the ground [where they] molt to the next stage . . . that of an eight-legged nymph. The nymph climbs up grass or plants and seeks another host in the same way as the larvae did. It remains attached for about five days and then drops to the ground to molt to the adult stage. The adult repeats the process, but only the females take a prolonged meal of blood, which lasts from eight to nine days. The males may attach lightly for a few hours, but their main concern is to find and mate with the females.*

It is when the tick is feeding that it transmits the germ of Lyme disease. Seventy to 90 percent of the people who contract Lyme disease are bitten by nymphs, which are much tinier than the adults. A nymph *Ixodes* is no larger than the period at the end of this sentence and may easily go unnoticed during a human feeding. Adults, on the other hand, are about as big as a pinhead or sesame seed and more easily detected. The female can bloat to the size of a pea after engorging with blood. The adults feed during early winter, the larvae during spring, and the nymphs during summer. The preferred or maintenance hosts are field mice and deer (or an occasional bear), giving *Ixodes* the name *deer tick*. However, nearly any warm-blooded animal will serve as an incidental host. Some fifty species of birds and thirty species of mammals have been implicated as hosts of *Ixodes* ticks, including household pets.

The Great Impostor

A person gets Lyme disease after being bitten by an infected deer tick. Other arthropods have been found to harbor *B. burgdorferi*, but ticks are the primary vector. The disease cannot be transmitted directly from one infected person to another. Lyme disease typically has three stages: (1) rash and flulike symptoms, (2) heart and nervous system disorders, (3) arthritis.

At stage 1, or primary Lyme, the rash appears at the bite location from several days to a month after the bite. It most often resembles a bull's-eye or target, with concentric red rings. It usually starts out small—two or three inches (five to eight centimeters) in diameter—but may expand to more than twenty inches (fifty-one centimeters) as the spirochetes invade surrounding tissue. The center of the target may fade and become clear. Along with the rash, the victim may experience a sore throat, fever, chills, fatigue, muscle ache, headache, joint swelling, and general flulike malaise.

If left untreated, about 20 percent of Lyme disease sufferers will develop acute heart and/or nervous system problems (stage 2, or secondary Lyme). The disease may mimic Bell's palsy, causing facial paralysis and pain. It may cause rapid or abnormal heartbeat (requiring a temporary pacemaker), light-headedness, difficulty breathing, migrainelike headaches, encephalitis, and meningitis. These conditions may last for weeks or months.

If the disease is still left untreated, about half of the sufferers will develop arthritis, usually in the knees (stage 3, or tertiary Lyme). The onset may be months or years after initial infection and may remain indefinitely. In worst-case scenarios, Lyme disease has also been known to damage the liver, eyes, kidneys, spleen, lungs, bone, and brain. It is believed that the spirochete can remain dormant in these tissues for many years, escaping antibiotic treatment, and then reactivate when the body's immune system becomes weakened.

Or Lyme disease may show none of the typical symptoms. The classic pattern of illness is not seen in many patients. One-third of Lyme disease sufferers do not even notice a rash, the most obvious indicator. The variability of symptoms makes it very difficult to diagnose the disease. It can mimic about eighty other illnesses. For this reason it has been called the "great impostor." Most commonly it is mistaken for the flu.

A four-and-a-half-year study conducted by Dr. Steere underscores the difficulty in accurately diagnosing the disease. Working at the New England

Medical Center, he studied 788 patients who were referred to the Lyme disease clinic at the center. Only 180 had active Lyme disease. In the study, 45 percent of the patients *without* Lyme disease had blood samples that tested positive. Blood tests are especially inaccurate for early diagnosis, since it may take six to eight weeks after a person is bitten by an infected tick for Lyme disease antibodies to show up. (Relatively new and sensitive immunological assays are being developed that can detect illness as early as one to two weeks after an infectious tick bite.)

Treatment

Lyme disease is not a killer (though it has been implicated in several deaths since its discovery). It can, however, cripple and cause permanent organ damage if left untreated. Treatment is generally successful with a number of broad-spectrum antibiotics taken orally, including the penicillins, tetracyclines, and cephalosporins. If left untreated until the third stage, hospitalization and intravenous antibiotic administration may be necessary. Its frequent misdiagnosis as the flu is especially unfortunate since that nearly always delays treatment. The flu is caused by a virus, and viral diseases are not treated with antibiotics. Lyme disease costs society more than one billion dollars every year from misdiagnoses that lead to expensive medical treatment and lost wages.

Prevention

There is one obvious way to prevent Lyme disease: don't get bitten by an infected tick. This is easier said than done. Many people live near wooded areas or enjoy hiking, camping, or other outdoor activities that place them in contact with hungry ticks and therefore at high risk. There are ways, however, to minimize this risk, most of which are common sense and easy to do. The CDC suggests the following, especially during tick season, which extends from April to October (though tick bites do occur year-round):

When walking through a wooded area or even across a lawn:
- Wear shoes and socks.
- Wear long pants cinched at the ankles or tucked into boots or socks.

- Wear light-colored clothing so that ticks will be easier to see.
- Use a repellent that is recommended for ticks (e.g., containing DEET).

When hiking or camping (in addition to the preceding rules):
- Stay in the middle of paths or trails, away from grass and shrubs.
- When setting up camp, use an insecticide on the surrounding area.

When gardening (in addition to the preceding rules):
- Wear gloves and a long-sleeved shirt.

Around your home:
- Treat the lawn with an insecticide specifically for ticks.
- Mow the lawn often. Ticks like tall grass (four inches—ten centimeters—or more). Short grass gets too dry and hot.

With pets:
- Check often for ticks.
- Bathe them regularly with a tick shampoo and use tick repellent and collars.

Over the past several years a vaccine against Lyme disease, called LYMErix, was developed. It was approved for use in the United States by the FDA on December 21, 1998, and marketed by the pharmaceutical giant SmithKline Beecham. Since its launch, the drug company says more than one million doses of LYMErix have been distributed to health departments, hospitals, doctors, and clinics. As of April 2002, however, SmithKline has discontinued distribution, citing poor sales.

But perhaps it is more than poor sales. LYMErix has had a checkered history since its approval. Although involved in a large-scale, premarketing efficacy study (11,000 people), in which it was deemed safe and about 85 percent effective, there is some indication that its active ingredient may trigger a nontreatable, crippling degenerative disease, autoimmune arthritis, in about one-third of the general population. A class-action lawsuit, *Karen Cassidy et al. v. SmithKline Beecham*, is pending, alleging that the drug company knew about and failed to warn doctors and the general public of the vaccine's potential hazard. Dr. Christine DeMarco, a member of the New Jersey Governor's Council on Lyme Disease, supports the plaintiffs in the legal action, while the FDA, the Health Commissioner of Duchess County (New York), Dr. Michael Caldwell, and both the New Jersey and New York State Departments of health cite the vaccine's safety and support its use—especially in cases when an individual is at high risk for contracting the disease. The vaccine, however, has not been tested in persons younger than fifteen years of age and is therefore not recommended for use in infants or children, even among its supporters—if and when it is remarketed.

A Lyme disease vaccine is available for dogs—with no anticipated legal action.

Distribution

In 1975 the first case of Lyme disease was discovered in a small rural town in Connecticut. Today it infects people in forty-eight U.S. states, in nineteen other countries, and on every continent except Antarctica. Within the United States the disease is most prevalent in the Northeast, upper Midwest, and coastal counties in California north of San Francisco, where large deer populations mix with dense human populations. (Since 1989, 75 percent of cases have been reported from just four northeastern states: New York, Connecticut, New Jersey, and Pennsylvania.) However, with the realization that migratory birds are acceptable hosts for the deer tick, it is expected that the disease will continue to spread to areas with a temperate climate.

Removing a Tick

Do not try to suffocate the tick by covering it with oil, petroleum jelly, nail polish remover, gasoline, or other poisonous chemicals. Never try to burn it off, and never squeeze its body. These methods, rather than removing the tick, cause it to burrow deeper into the skin and to regurgitate spirochetes. Instead, grasp the tick as close to the skin as possible using tweezers or forceps and pull upward in a slow, steady motion. Removing an infected tick from the skin within twenty-four hours greatly reduces the risk of contracting the disease.

After removal, disinfect and dress the bitten area. Save the tick to show your doctor. If you develop any symptoms of Lyme disease or the flu within a month after being bitten, see your doctor. If you are pregnant, see your doctor immediately. Though the disease is not transmitted from person to person, the bacterium can pass from mother to fetus across the placenta.

Imitating the Great Impostor

Within the past decade, another tick-borne disease has emerged from the bushes and made its way into the headlines: human granulocytic ehrlichiosis (HGE), or ehrlichia. It was first recognized in the midwestern United States in 1993 and since then has spread to the Northeast. Nearly one thousand confirmed and probable cases have been reported as of 2000, but experts believe there are many more that go unreported or are being misdiagnosed as Lyme disease. HGE is caused by a bacterium that is different from the one responsible for Lyme disease.

The symptoms of HGE are very similar to those of Lyme except that there is no telltale rash. The onset of the disease is quicker and its effects more acute; and unlike Lyme, it can be deadly, with a fatality rate approaching 5 percent. Treatment with antibiotics, if begun within ten to fourteen days of the first symptoms, is generally effective. Unlike Lyme, which responds to a range of antibiotics, HGE is standardly treated only with tetracycline and one of its relatives, doxycycline. (Oral doxycycline is usually not prescribed for children until after all their permanent teeth have erupted; it can permanently discolor teeth that are still forming.)

Presently, there is no vaccine for ehrlichia as there is for Lyme disease, and the most effective prevention is to limit one's exposure to ticks.

The Flesh Eaters

A man living in Toronto nicks his finger while sharpening a pair of ice skates. An infection develops in the wound; the infection quickly moves up his arm. The man feels ill for several days and goes to the hospital complaining of fever, vomiting, and swollen lymph nodes in his armpit. He is examined, given medication, and sent home. A day later he is readmitted to the hospital, deathly ill. In less than twenty-four hours the infection has literally eaten away all of the flesh and muscle on his upper arm, shoulder, and back. By the following day the man is dead.

A seventy-one-year-old woman living in New York City nicks her leg while shaving. The following day the leg is swollen, and the day after that she must be hospitalized. The leg is gangrenous, the flesh eaten away. It must be amputated. The woman never wakes up from surgery—she is dead in four days as a result of a superficial razor cut.

These people did not die in the Middle Ages or even in the early part of this century, before the age of antibiotics. They died in 1995! What killed them was the same germ that up to 30 percent of the population carries harmlessly on their skin and that occasionally causes a mild sore throat. They died of strep.

Chains of Death

Streptococci are Gram-positive spherical bacteria that grow in chains, like a string of pearls. As they grow, they secrete toxins and enzymes. Depending on how certain of these chemicals damage red blood cells, streptococci are classified as alpha(α)-hemolytic, beta(β)-hemolytic, or gamma(γ)-hemolytic. The category that concerns us is β-hemolytic.

Strep germs are further differentiated into groups A through O, based on the nature of certain chemicals attached to their cell wall. The group that concerns us is A. Our villain is, therefore, β-hemolytic group A streptococcus, or *group A strep* for short.

There are more than eighty different strains of group A strep. Depending on the strain and the vulnerability of the human host, they can cause a wide variety of diseases. In fact, the strep A bacterium is responsible for more human diseases than any other. The mildest of these are ordinary sore throats, skin rashes, and skin lesions called *impetigo*. More serious afflictions include strep throats, scarlet fever, rheumatic fever, and childbed fever. Before the era of antibiotics, scarlet and childbed fever were epidemic killers. During the American Civil War, strep A infections were a major cause of death. And they still are in third-world countries, where living conditions are poor and health care inadequate. In developed nations, with the use of antibiotics, they are no longer a serious threat.

All group A strep infections are sensitive to antibiotics. They have not developed resistance to the old-timer penicillin, as many infections have, and there is no hint yet that they will start. They have, however, shown resistance to the next drug of choice for those who are allergic to penicillin—streptomycin. A newer drug, clindamycin, has proved surprisingly effective against strep A, especially when treatment is delayed, and no resistance to clindamycin has been indicated thus far.

A few strains, however, have become extremely aggressive, producing powerful toxins and enzymes that can cause death before antibiotics have a chance to work. These extremely aggressive types are known collectively as *invasive group A strep* (*IGAS*) and include those with a taste for human flesh.

Statistics

IGAS came into prominence in early 1994, when fifteen people in Britain contracted the flesh-eating form and eleven of them died. The tabloids grabbed hold of it and ran front-page headlines such as "KILLER BUG ATE MY FACE," with pictures of victims that could have come straight out of a horror flick. The world was thrown into a panic.

Cooler heads eventually prevailed. The disease is not epidemic; it does not threaten humanity. It is also a disease that scientists have known about for a while. IGAS was first described in 1924. The flesh-eating form was well known during World War II but then disappeared until the mid-1980s. It is likely that the germ returned with greater virulence. Dr. P. Patrick Cleary, a microbiologist at the University of Minnesota, discovered that some invasive strep bacteria acquired a viral infection around 1987. (For a full discussion of these strange "bugs" called viruses, see Chapter 6.) He speculates that the virus gave them powerful toxin-producing genes.

According to studies conducted by the CDC, invasive strep infects ten to fifteen thousand people in the United States annually (garden-variety strep infects millions). Of these, five hundred to fifteen hundred are flesh-eaters. Flesh-eating strep kills about 20 percent of the people who contract it, or one hundred to three hundred people each year. Invasive strep, overall, kills two to three thousand Americans each year. Not common, but significant.

IGAS has also killed people in many countries other than the United States and Great Britain, including Canada, Europe, and third-world nations.

A Deadly Cut

The disease is generally contracted through a break in the skin, which becomes infected with the invasive strep microbe. A nick from shaving, a thorn prick while gardening, a paper cut, a hangnail, is all it takes. An eight-year-old boy in New York City got the infection through a chicken pox sore and died three days later. People have contracted IGAS after C-section and vaginal births, after scratching a rash, after a friendly punch in the arm, from having blood drawn during a routine physical exam, or from surgery. Or from no known invasive procedure or trauma at all. People who have strep throats or other strep infections are more susceptible because they are already harboring a related infection and risk contracting the more virulent IGAS through reinfection (such as from coughing into their hand and then touching an open wound). The possibility of harboring aggressive strep in a population of garden-variety strep is always there. Also, the elderly are more susceptible, as are those who have been ill recently or who are on immunosuppressant drugs, because of their compromised immune systems.

Once the wound has become infected with IGAS, the disease progresses with amazing rapidity. The flesh-eating form can destroy human tissue at the rate of an inch (2.5 centimeters) an hour. Victims literally see their flesh being "devoured." Flesh-eating group A strep infections have been given the fancy name *necrotizing fasciitis*. If the germ has a preference for muscle tissue, the disease is called *necrotizing myositis* (*myo* means "muscle"). In most cases the bug just eats—or, more accurately, dissolves—whatever is around: muscle, flesh, organs.

The germ does not always kill by eating away tissue. If the toxins it produces enter the bloodstream, they may kill by causing the victim to go into shock—a generalized response that includes a drastic drop in blood pressure, raging fever, and organ failure. The complex set of symptoms is known collectively as *toxic shock syndrome*, or *TSS*. In 1990 Jim Henson, creator of the Muppets, died of TSS, induced by aggressive group A strep toxins. The fatality rate of streptococcal TSS is as high as 60 percent. (A very similar condition afflicted women in the late seventies and early eighties. In those cases, however, the cause of TSS was not strep, but another common bug turned deadly, our old enemy *Staphylococcus aureus*—the stuff of boils. Women using superabsorbent tampons were contracting the infection vaginally.)

The problem with treating IGAS infections is that they kill so quickly. This is compounded by the fact that they can be easily misdiagnosed. (Symptoms of necrotizing fasciitis resemble the "flu," and its effects on the flesh can, early on, be indistinguishable from acute cellulitis.) Antibiotics are effective against them, but they can take up to forty-eight hours to kick in. By that time it may be too late; the disease can kill within hours. Also, to be effective, antibiotics must be able to circulate and reach diseased tissue. In necrotizing fasciitis, the destroyed tissue has little or no blood circulation. Antibiotics cannot penetrate it to combat the infection. Ultimately, tissue destruction continues, poisons continue to be released, and the victim dies of organ damage or toxic shock. For this reason it is often necessary to remove the diseased and dead tissue surgically, which may involve limb amputation—after which broad-spectrum antibiotics are usually administered intravenously for seven days or longer.

Time Is of the Essence

It may be difficult to prevent IGAS infection, which can happen with the simplest break in the skin. If possible, wash, disinfect, and dress the wound as quickly as possible. Bleeding of the wound is also desirable in that it helps prevent germs from entering the body. It is a natural wash. Once infection has occurred, vigilance and quick action are the operative words. If the area surrounding the wound reddens or becomes swollen—and especially if it increases in size—or if fever or flulike symptoms develop, see a doctor immediately. Do not delay. Waiting just a day can be half a day too late. Though the disease is relatively rare, it can kill.

Prevention

Dr. Vincent Fischetti, a Brooklyn-born microbiologist, has been doing battle with streptococcus for some forty years. He is known affectionately as Dr. Strep. Several years ago, in a remarkable breakthrough, he discovered a vaccine that has proved effective in preventing strep infections in laboratory animals. As of May 2002, the vaccine is in human clinical trials; it has been tested in more than one hundred volunteers and deemed to be safe. The vaccine takes advantage of the fact that streptococcus—in fact, Gram-positive bacteria in general, which include the deadly staph, pneumococcus, and clostridium—uses molecules on its surface to invade tissues. It is its mode of pathogenicity. Dr. Fischetti has developed a vaccine that interferes with the proper attachment of the bacterium to its host. When placed into the nasopharynx of mice, it remained there for up to twelve weeks, producing antibodies. If successful, the world may soon be rid of flesh-eating strep, the strep that causes toxic shock, and the broad range of strep infections that continue to kill tens of thousands of people worldwide—many of them children. It may also prove an effective prophylaxis against a wide band of other infectious diseases.

As a sidebar, Dr. Fischetti and his team at the Rockefeller University have isolated an enzyme that kills the "bioterror bug" anthrax, which is in the early stages of clinical trials.

Legionnaires' Disease: Opportunity Knocks

On July 21, 1976, twenty-five hundred delegates of the Pennsylvania Department of the American Legion, along with two thousand family members and friends, assembled in Philadelphia to celebrate the two-hundredth anniversary of America's Declaration of Independence. They attended meetings and banquets, conducted business, and partied. After four days the bicentennial convention ended, and they dispersed to different parts of the state to resume their everyday lives. Within several weeks thirty-four of them would be dead from a mysterious form of pneumonia that would come to be known as *Legionnaires' disease.*

Hunt for a Killer

Because the victims had dispersed to dozens of towns and villages across the state before showing symptoms of the disease, a connection between the convention and the pneumonia outbreak was not made until a week after the convention had ended. On August 2 the state health department was notified and an alert was issued. The CDC in Atlanta was also called in. Twelve people were already dead from the disease, which typically ran the following course (some of these symptoms may not occur):

1. General malaise (flulike symptoms): loss of appetite, muscle pains, headache, low-grade fever
2. Chest and abdominal pains, diarrhea, nausea
3. Spike in fever—up to 105°F (41°C)—with shaking chills
4. Dry cough
5. Pneumonia
6. Mental confusion or delirium

The kidneys and liver were also commonly involved. In extreme cases a patient would have to be placed on an artificial kidney due to renal failure. Incubation of the disease was from two to ten days, and illness lasted for seven to ten days. In total, 1 in 6.5 patients died (221 people developed the disease). Curiously, men were about three times more susceptible than women. Smokers, alcoholics, the elderly, and those who were ill or in some way immunocompromised were also at greater risk. Hospitals would become a favored place for contracting the disease.

The Bellevue-Stratford Hotel was heavily suspected as the source of infection at the Philadelphia convention. All of the people who got ill had either stayed at the hotel, visited it, or passed along the street directly in front of it. But the questions remained: what was the cause of the disease, and how were people contracting it?

An infectious disease can be gotten in one of several ways: it can be transmitted from person to person, through an arthropod or other animal bite, or ingested with food or water. It can enter through a break in the skin or through thin mucous lining—as in certain sexually transmitted diseases. In the case of Legionnaires' disease, person-to-person transmission was quickly ruled out. After the initial outbreak the disease did not spread. Pest bites were also ruled out; they did not fit the pattern of the disease. The food and water served at the Bellevue-Stratford were tested on laboratory animals; they did not cause the disease either.

The CDC then began testing lung tissue from dead Legionnaires for possible pathogens. The pathology department made thin slices of the tissue, colored them with stains, and then stuck them under the microscope. No microbes were found. The bacteriology department spread the lung tissue on culture plates with fourteen different kinds of growth media. Nothing grew.

These negative findings caused the investigators to suspect a virus. Viruses are very small and difficult to see—you need an electron microscope—and they do not grow on culture plates; they need living cells. Sections of lung tissue were therefore given to the virology department, where small bits were inoculated into live chick eggs. Nothing grew—except the chicks.

With increasing desperation, the CDC researchers expanded their search to unlikely areas. They gave samples of lung tissue to the rickettsia department. Rickettsia are like viruses in that they require living hosts and are difficult to see under a microscope, but they are bacteria. Rickettsia cause Rocky Mountain spotted fever, typhus, and a disease called Q *fever*. But they did not cause Legionnaires' disease.

At this point focus turned from biological to chemical causes. Perhaps the culprit was a toxic substance, like mercury or lead. There are about thirty metallic elements and thirty-five thousand organic compounds that are toxic to living systems. Extensive testing by toxicologists on both fronts proved negative.

After months of exhaustive work and at a cost of about two million dollars, the world's top disease detectives had failed to uncover the Legionnaire killer. Their disappointment was compounded by an unsympathetic press, which hinted at a broad-based cover-up or possibly sabotage. Staten Island, New York, Congressman John M. Murphy was especially critical, charging it was unfathomable that in a country "with the most advanced technology in the world, we find ourselves in a position of not knowing what happened in Philadelphia." He went so far as to suggest that an antimilitary fanatic had somehow murdered the Legionnaires.

The CDC published a report in mid-December 1976 summarizing its abortive investigation. Among those who read the report was Dr. Joseph McDade, the scientist who had tested the diseased lung tissue samples for rickettsia several months earlier. Though he had not found any, he did notice a few rod-shaped bacteria on his slides, which he dismissed at the time as insignificant or unrelated. He was no longer so sure.

Reexamining his slides more carefully, he found many more rod-shaped microbes. Next he performed serological tests to confirm that they were indeed the cause of Legionnaires' disease. He mixed the blood of patients who had contracted the disease and built up antibodies against it with cultures of his suspect bacteria. The antibodies in the blood attached to the bac-

teria in a typical immune response. McDade had found the smoking gun—
and the bullet in the body as well. It turned out to be an entirely new organism, genus as well as species, which was rare. They named the bullet
Legionella pneumophila (pneumophila means "lung-loving" in Greek), and
Legionnaires' disease was officially dubbed *legionellosis*. It was January 1977.

Subsequent studies with *L. pneumophila* uncovered the reasons why
the CDC microbe hunters were unable to see it or grow it. It is an extraor-
dinarily fastidious organism. It will not color and become visible with ordinary stains and will not grow on ordinary media. Investigators were
eventually able to stain the beast with a yellow dye developed more than
sixty years ago for the spirochete that causes syphilis. They were eventually able to grow it by adding a truckload of iron and the amino acid cysteine to their media. For some reason *L. pneumophila* is an iron and
cysteine junkie. Also, it was learned that mice do not get Legionnaires' disease; they have a natural immunity. Guinea pigs are not so lucky. The use
of mice as test animals certainly hampered the investigation.

Out of the Mist

After *L. pneumophila* was identified as the causative agent of Legionnaires'
disease, investigators returned their attention to the Bellevue-Stratford
Hotel. Where was the germ coming from? It was not in the food or water;
they had already been tested. A break came when certain workers at the
CDC remembered an outbreak of a similar though much milder disease
that had occurred eight years earlier, in the building of the county health
department at Pontiac, Michigan. Ninety-five out of a hundred people
working in the building had come down with "Pontiac fever," which produces flulike symptoms but not pneumonia. The cause of the disease was
never determined, but an evaporative condenser that was part of the air-
conditioning system of the building was heavily implicated. Guinea pigs
made to breathe a mist from the condenser developed Pontiac fever. The
CDC was unable to isolate an organism or chemical substance from the
mist, but it did store blood from the human victims.

Eight years later this blood was taken out of frozen storage, thawed,
and put through serological tests with *L. pneumophila*. The blood contained antibodies against Legionnaires' disease. *L. pneumophila* was also
the cause of Pontiac fever. This confirmation led the CDC bloodhounds to

the air-conditioning system at the Bellevue-Stratford. It was, at the time, determined to be the source of the bicentennial outbreak of Legionnaires' in the city of brotherly love. New data, however, suggest that the water in the hotel—originally eliminated as a suspect—was the actual culprit.

L. pneumophila has since been found in showerheads, steam turbines, hot tubs, whirlpool spas, steam rooms, fountains, grocery store vegetable misters, and plain old water pipes. It has been found in natural environments: ponds, slow-flowing creeks, hot springs, stagnant lakes, and their surrounding banks. The bacterium becomes particularly dangerous when it is airborne and can be breathed in. According to the website Legionella.org, "The major source [of infection] is water distribution systems of large buildings, including hotels and hospitals. Cooling towers have long been thought to be a major source for *Legionella*, but new data suggest that this is an overemphasized mode of transmission. Air conditioners are not a source for Legionnaires' disease."

To prevent *L. pneumophila* from collecting, all devices that hold water or release it into the atmosphere should be cleaned regularly with a disinfectant. *L. pneumophila* is especially resistant to chlorine. Water treatment facilities routinely chlorinate water at .2 part per million. To kill *L. pneumophila*, a concentration ten times that is necessary. Also, the microbe can survive in temperatures up to 130°F (54°C). It is capable of living for more than a year inside water pipes in thin biofilms and then emerging fully infectious once the tap is turned on. Stagnant water provides a breeding ground for the organism.

An Opportunist

It is likely that *Legionella* has been around for some time, perhaps hundreds of years. Yet Legionnaires' disease seems to be a recent arrival—a contemporary killer. The earliest known cases occurred in 1947, which is little more than fifty years ago. Why hasn't it shown itself much earlier, as have the vast majority of infectious diseases?

Perhaps it has. It is likely that Legionnaires' disease was frequently misdiagnosed as the flu or nonspecific pneumonia. The difficulty in seeing and growing *Legionella* did not help. These reasons notwithstanding, the disease seems to have exploded as a twentieth-century phenomenon. Why?

Technology, my dear Watson. According to Bernard Dixon in *Power Unseen*, *L. pneumophila* is "an opportunist *par excellence*, capable of living unnoticed in locations such as cooling towers, humidifiers [now disclaimed somewhat], and showers, which causes potentially fatal disease when it is released into the air as a mist or aerosol." Things that mist water are largely products of modern technology—the age of electronics. They provided *Legionella* with an effective mode of entry into the body and added another killer to the long list of human pathogens.*

Unlike many other infectious diseases, Legionnaires' is more prevalent in developed rather than developing nations. Aside from Pontiac and Philadelphia, outbreaks have occurred throughout the United States as well as in Great Britain and Europe. In July 1994 one occurred aboard a luxury cruise liner, *Horizon*, owned by Celebrity Cruise Lines. *L. pneumophila* was found in the water system of the fifteen-hundred-passenger ship that cruises to Bermuda and the Caribbean. Three passengers died of the disease.

According to health and science writer Laurie Garrett, "The CDC estimated that somewhere between 2,000 and 6,000 people had been dying every year of Legionnaires' disease, probably for decades, certainly since the advent of air-conditioning technology. Prior to the dramatic Philadelphia outbreak, these cases had simply been dumped into the category of 'pneumonia of unknown etiology' " (*The Coming Plague*). An estimated eight thousand to eighteen thousand Americans develop Legionnaires' annually according to the CDC. However, as with many diseases that are not clearly distinguishable from other diseases, the actual incidence may be significantly higher. Other sources have estimated as many as one hundred thousand annual cases in the United States.

Two Faces of Legionella

It is somewhat puzzling that the same organism is responsible for both the deadly Legionnaires' diseases and the much milder Pontiac fever, which never kills, has a much shorter incubation period, and doesn't cause pneumonia—the classic symptom of Legionnaires' disease. The damage caused by the microbe is related to the enzymes it produces, and there are about

---

*According to legionella.org (January 25, 2002): "The most popular theory is that the organism is aerosolized in water and people inhale the droplets containing *Legionella*. However, new evidence suggests that . . . 'aspiration' is the most common way that bacteria enter into the lungs to cause pneumonia. Aspiration means choking such that secretions in the mouth get past the choking reflexes and instead of going into the esophagus and stomach, mistakenly enter the lungs."

thirty-five species of *Legionella* presently known to be pathogenic, with dozens of strains within each species. Perhaps certain of these produce enzymes that are considerably more destructive than others.

Both diseases are treatable with antibiotic drugs. During an outbreak of Legionnaires' disease in Burlington, Vermont, in 1977, doctors treated cases with a range of antibiotics. Erythromycin, a member of a class of drugs called *macrolides*, was found to be the most effective—much more so than penicillin—as the "Legion killer." It was the drug of choice for many years. Recently, it has been replaced with more effective, less toxic macrolides (for example, azithromycin) and another class of antibiotics, the quinolones (for example, ciprofloxacin—"Cipro" of anthrax fame—and levofloxacin). Rifampin, of tuberculosis fame, has also been used as a secondary drug in stubborn cases.

Legionnaires' has a mortality rate ranging typically from 5 to 20 percent, according to the Canadian Centre for Occupational Health and Safety. However, this rate is population-sensitive. A CDC study of reported cases indicated a death rate of 40 percent for cases acquired during a hospital stay (nosocomial cases), where patient resistance and general health are lower.

General health does not dictate only death rate but also risk of infection. People who are immunocompromised or in poor health increase this risk. According to a health-information website, hcinfo.com, "HIV-infected patients . . . have a 40-fold increased risk; organ transplant recipients have a 200-fold increased risk. Smokers, persons over 65 years of age and heavy drinkers have a moderately higher risk." Add to this list diabetics, asthmatics, cancer patients—virtually anyone suffering a debilitating condition. And though the numbers may vary, the concept applies not only to Legionnaires' disease but to infection in general.

6

The Virus

Nothing brings us so close to the riddle of Life—and to its solution—as viruses.

—WOLFHARD WEIDEL

IN SEVENTEENTH-CENTURY Holland people paid fantastic sums of money to decorate their gardens with tulips that were not solid in color but streaked in a random, paint-splashed manner. It was a phenomenon known as *color-breaking* in tulips, and it became the craze. Wealthy men offered homes, farms, even their daughters in marriage for a single color-variegated bulb. The cause of such natural beauty? A virus.

In Zaire a man feels a throbbing behind his eyeballs. It is January 8, 1980. Several days later his eyeballs turn bright red. Within a week he begins bleeding profusely from every orifice of his body. Blood pours from his mouth, nose, anus, eyes, ears. Even his nipples bleed. Along with the blood come sloughed-off intestines and esophagus linings. The man is literally liquefying of an incurable hemorrhagic disease called *Ebola*. The cause? A virus.

On April 18, 1993, pulmonary specialist Ron Crystal at the National Institutes of Health in Bethesda, Maryland, snakes a flexible tube called a *bronchoscope* down the throat of a cystic fibrosis patient. Cystic fibrosis (CF) is a devastating genetic disorder that causes the lungs and digestive organs to clog with a thick, sticky mucus. This mucus is a breeding ground for bacteria. Most CF sufferers die of lung disease or heart failure by their early thirties.

The bronchoscope is supposed to drip a fluid into the man's lungs. It is a fluid that contains millions of copies of a normal gene with which to correct the defective cells of the lungs. The technology, called *gene therapy*, is cutting edge. What will deliver these life-saving genes into the pulmonary cells? A virus.

Viruses are the tiniest of all living things. Bacteria, small one-celled organisms that can be seen only under a light microscope, are huge compared to viruses. A single drop of blood can contain six billion viruses, a number greater than the human population of Earth. Small wonder the existence of viruses was not even suspected until the beginning of the twentieth century. And it was not until 1939, with the invention of the powerful electron microscope, that the first virus was actually seen. Since then we have learned much about what viruses are and what they do.

The Discovery of Viruses

Although viruses have probably been around since life on this planet began, they were discovered only a scant hundred years ago. In 1892 a Russian botanist, Dmitry Ivanovsky, was investigating tobacco mosaic disease, which caused mottling and blistering of tobacco leaves. It was an affliction that threatened the tobacco industry of Russia and Europe. Ivanovsky passed the sap of infected plants through a porcelain filter that was believed to trap all types of microorganisms, including bacteria, the smallest known pathogens. The filter had been invented by Charles Chamberlain, the trusted assistant of Louis Pasteur, and was used in many homes to filter and purify drinking water.

Surprisingly, however, the filtered sap still caused infection. Obviously the infectious agent was making it through the filter. Could the disease be caused by a poison or toxin made by the bacteria? Certain human diseases such as diphtheria were indeed caused by potent bacterial toxins that would easily pass through Chamberlain filters. Many scientists believed this to be the case. Alas, they were mistaken.

A half dozen years later another botanist, this time a Dutchman named Martinus Beijerinck, continued the investigation. He took the sap from an infected plant, sprayed it on a healthy plant, took the sap from that plant after it became diseased, and in this manner passed the sap through several plant generations. Through all the successive inoculations plants continued to develop the characteristic mottling of tobacco mosaic disease. The sap retained its full virulence after any number of plant passages. This nondilutable property suggested an entity that was reproducing itself within the plant. So much for the idea of toxins.

Strange happenings. It wasn't a bacterium, and it wasn't a toxin. At first Beijerinck called the infectious agent a *contagium vivium fluidum*— a "contagious living fluid." Later he coined the term *virus*, which is Latin for "poison" or "poisonous slime." Still, no one really knew what they were dealing with. In many ways, as HIV and other emerging viruses so cruelly demonstrate, they still don't.

Lack of knowledge about the nature of viruses notwithstanding, soon other diseases were found to be caused by this "soluble living germ." Foot-and-mouth disease of cattle was the first animal illness shown to be transmitted by a filterable agent smaller than any known bacterium. By 1900 a human disease, yellow fever, was proved to be of viral origin. Today we know of thousands of different viruses, and they infect everything that is alive. But as the twentieth century dawned, scientists had hardly passed the point of asking, "Couldn't a virus be merely a supertiny bacterium that can make it through a filter?"

How Do Viruses Work?

No, viruses are not supertiny bacteria. Viruses and bacteria are, in fact, so fundamentally different that in many respects a bacterium is more closely related to a human than to a virus. At least humans and bacteria are both made of cells. All living things are cellular except viruses. The structures within a cell necessary to perform the life activities of eating, energy production, growth, and response to environmental change are absent in a virus. A virus is, in fact, nothing more than a tiny, lifeless, totally inert particle—as long as it remains outside the cell. Tragically it is made to get inside the cell. Once inside, the deadly game of viral infection begins.

To understand how a virus does its thing, we must take a closer look at this obligate intracellular parasite. All viruses consist of two parts: a nucleic acid core and a protein coat surrounding the core. In some cases there is an additional fatty, or lipid, envelope. It is the function of the protein coat and lipid envelope (if present) to attach the viral particle to the cell membrane and—somehow—get the virus into the cell. This is not easy. The surface of the viral coat must fit exactly into "receptor" sites on the cell membrane. If the fit is not precise, then attachment and subsequent penetration into the cell cannot occur. Even in an ideal matchup probably only one out of every few thousand encounters between virus and suitable cell results in proper binding of the two. The exactness of fit necessary for viral binding or attachment explains why viruses are usually species-specific—they will not infect cells of totally different species. Notable exceptions are the rabies and influenza viruses, both of which have a wide range of hosts.

Not only will viruses seldom infect totally different species, but quite often they are specific to particular types of cells within an organism. The hepatitis B virus targets liver cells. HIV goes for particular binding sites, or markers, on certain white blood cells. Viruses that cause the common cold bind to cells lining the respiratory tract.

Once the virus is attached to the cell, it can penetrate the membrane and enter the cell in a number of ways. It may cause the cell membrane to infold and pinch off a tiny vesicle with the virus inside. Viruses with fatty envelopes may fuse their envelopes with the cell membrane, penetrating it and letting the rest of the virus into the cell.

By whatever means, when a virus gets inside the cell, it can do one of several things. What it does determines the course of the disease. In many cases the virus begins replicating itself immediately. Reproduction and widespread distribution are, after all, a virus's raison d'être. To accomplish this the virus commandeers the machinery of the cell, coercing it into churning out more viral particles. It is an incredible act of piracy that is orchestrated and controlled by the virus's nucleic acid.

Nucleic acid is a remarkable substance whose biological importance was not realized until 1953. It was in that year that James Watson and

Francis Crick determined the molecular structure of DNA, one type of nucleic acid. There is another type, called RNA. If we are to understand the workings of viruses, we must first understand DNA and RNA.

DNA is the substance of genes—the genetic material. Found in every living cell (except mature red blood cells), it is what makes a tree a tree, a bacterium a bacterium, and a human a human. It is what makes one human different from another. Structurally speaking, DNA can be viewed as a very, very long, microscopic charm bracelet (three billion charms in the case of humans). More accurately, it is two charm bracelets, lined up so that their charms bond to one another. There are four different kinds of charms, called nitrogen bases and designated by the letters A, T, C, and G. The double chain also has an obvious twist, giving it the overall look of a twisted rope ladder (a double helix), with the rungs representing the paired nitrogen bases.

Like a four-letter alphabet, the sequence of rungs or base pairs spells out what a cell will do and become. It is a blueprint for life, controlling the functioning of a cell by determining the proteins that the cell makes. But DNA does not work alone. It does not, in fact, directly control protein synthesis, which occurs on tiny particles, or protein factories, that float around the cell. DNA lies buried deep within the nucleus, interwoven into the fabric of the chromosomes like Madame Defarge's secrets. It is too valuable to go traipsing around the cell. Instead, it makes a messenger strand of nucleic acid using its base pair sequence as a template. This messenger molecule is RNA, and it carries the code from the DNA to the protein factories outside the nucleus.

Now back to our obligate intracellular parasite. Like living cells, viruses contain nucleic acid as their genetic material. A particular virus may contain DNA or RNA but not both. Unlike the DNA of the cell, however, viral nucleic acid codes not for cellular proteins but for proteins necessary to make more viruses. And it forces the cell to do just that—churn out proteins that the virus needs to make more of itself. It is an ingenious multiphased takeover that goes something like this:

1. Proteins are produced that are predominantly enzymatic in nature. They encourage reactions that produce many thousands of copies of viral nucleic acid.

2. After viral nucleic acid is synthesized, the structural coat proteins are produced.
3. The virus is assembled by having the coat protein form as a shell around the nucleic acid core.
4. These new viral particles are released, sometimes—but not always—killing the cell in the process. In some instances the virus grabs a snippet of cell membrane, which becomes its lipid envelope.

The precise mechanism by which viruses initiate their replication depends on the genetic material of the virus. A DNA virus, as some might expect, has a mode of action very similar to host DNA. First, a viral RNA is produced using the virus's DNA as a template. Then the RNA directs production of viral proteins. It can be summarized as follows: viral DNA → viral RNA → viral protein.

With most RNA viruses the first step is eliminated and the viral nucleic acid simply proceeds to make the proper viral proteins: viral RNA → viral protein.

The concept that DNA begets RNA, which begets protein is so basic to biology that it has come to be known as the *central dogma*. Never does RNA produce DNA. Never, that is, except in the case of a retrovirus. This class of RNA viruses, which counts HIV, the AIDS virus, among its members, startled molecular biologists by doing the unthinkable—by working backward. Instead of making protein, the retrovirus's RNA first goes in reverse and acts as a template for DNA synthesis. The DNA then makes another RNA, which finally goes about churning out protein molecules:

viral RNA → viral DNA → viral RNA → viral protein

Strange indeed, but, much to our misfortune, it works eminently well for the retrovirus. (More on this in Chapter 10, "AIDS.")

Acute Viral Infections

When a virus begins reproducing itself immediately and aggressively, an acute infection results. This is virus-host interaction at its simplest, and it is a common course for many viruses. Measles, mumps, meningitis, influenza, and the common cold are diseases in which infection is acute and the conflict lively between virus and immune system. When viral infection is acute, there is a head-on collision between virus and body defenses. Recovery from illness means complete elimination of the virus. An aggressive immune response is what makes vaccination against many acute diseases possible. A vaccine contains a germ that has been killed or made weak by heat or chemicals. Its similarity to the real virus or bacterium tricks the immune system into a vigorous response that can last a lifetime.

Acute infection, however, is not always the way in which a virus interacts with its host. In fact we are discovering that acute infection is not the norm. And why should it be? The more aggressively a virus reproduces within host cells and spreads to new cells, the more rapidly it kills its host. From the virus's point of view, this is not good, for without a host viruses cannot live. A virus would much rather live within an organism and cause that organism little or no harm.

This seems to be what the older, more well-established viruses tend to do. Over time and many generations they adapt to their hosts, becoming less virulent and allowing their meal tickets to survive. Even the common cold was a deadly killer five thousand years ago, when it was a recent arrival on the human scene. It is new viruses that wreak havoc on a population. And, oh, what havoc those ill-adapted viruses can wreak. As mentioned already, viruses brought to the New World by Columbus and Cortés enabled their armies to conquer the Amerindians. Native Americans might have waged battle successfully against the swords of the conquistadores but were no match for their smallpox microbes. In Mexico City between 1520 and 1522, three to four million Aztecs succumbed to new diseases of the Spanish invaders. Smallpox, measles, and influenza quite literally wiped out the Amerindians, with kill rates running as high as 95 percent in some cities.

Today we see the same thing happening when new viruses emerge from the rain forests and invade naive (never before exposed) populations. Ebola is a classic and chilling example. When it first emerged in 1976 in Zaire, it swept through fifty villages, killing in a most horrible manner over 90 percent of the people it infected.

Thankfully Ebola did not become a worldwide pandemic. Perhaps this was because its infection was so acute, often killing victims within a week.

Such rapid death did not allow hosts to spread the deadly microbes. With no living cells available, the fragile Ebola viruses withered away and died.

In a sense the Ebola virus brought about its own demise. A preferable course of action for viruses is one in which they engage not in heated combat with their hosts but rather in guerrilla warfare. Such hit-and-hide behavior successfully perpetuates the virus for many years within host cells and leads to what are termed *persistent infections*.

Persistent Viral Infections

People suffering from herpes simplex 1 and herpes simplex 2 infections are familiar with persistent viral infections. The word *herpes* comes from the Greek verb "to creep" and aptly describes the spreading lesions that characterize these related diseases.

Herpes simplex 1 attacks skin and mucous membrane cells of the mouth and lips, producing common cold sores. The simplex 2 virus infects similar cells of the genitalia, resulting in blistering. When these sores and blisters appear, viruses are actively multiplying and spreading to neighboring cells. Eventually antibodies stem the tide and neutralize the invading microbes. A crusty scab forms, and the battle is won—but not the war. The enemy has not been completely destroyed. Some viral particles manage to retreat to clumps of nerve cells in the face and neck called *ganglia*. Here they safely hide within the cells, well beyond the reach of the immune system, until some external stimulus or weakening of immunity reactivates the infection.

The hiding of a virus within body cells, totally undetected, is called *latency*. It is a trick that herpesviruses have mastered. When a virus is latent, it becomes completely dormant. The viral genes are present within host cells, but they do not express themselves. No viral proteins and no viral particles are produced.

Latent viruses can remain in this dormant state for many years, causing no symptoms in the host. Varicella-zoster, another virus in the herpesvirus family, demonstrates this long-term latency. In young children it produces the rash and fever of chicken pox. The immune system, called immediately into action, pounces hard on the virus and eliminates the infection. But varicella-zoster is a herpesvirus. Some of its viral particles escape destruction and retreat to ganglia of the vertebrae. Here the virus lies low, usually remaining dormant and never reactivating. Sometimes, however, for reasons we do not truly understand, the virus reemerges and begins replicating in nerve cells that run along the back. It tends to do so in older people and produces the painful rash of the disease called *shingles*.

With the discovery of latency, scientists have come to an unnerving realization: every single human being has viruses hidden within at least some of his or her body cells—viruses that can cause disease at any time. This point was illustrated most tragically in the highly publicized case of David, a child who was born with a rare genetic disorder. (He was the subject of a 1976 made-for-TV movie, *The Boy in the Plastic Bubble*.) David had no functioning immune system and had to live in a germ-free environment to prevent fatal infections. In the early 1980s he received a bone-marrow transplant from his sister in an attempt to establish an immune system. Unbeknownst to his physicians, however, the Epstein-Barr virus lay hidden within his sister's bone-marrow cells. Today we know that 90 percent of all people worldwide carry this virus, which, when active, is responsible for a not-too-serious disease called mononucleosis (the "kissing disease"). In David's defenseless body, however, the Epstein-Barr virus ran hog-wild, ravaging him with cancer—his intestine, liver, and brain became riddled with tumors. Within four months he died.

Yes, viruses cause cancer. It is one of the nastier consequences of some persistent viral infections. Today's medical researchers believe that 20 percent of all cancers are viral in origin. Most liver cancers result from infection with the hepatitis B virus. Several leukemias are initiated by viruses that are similar to HIV. Virtually all cervical cancers are associated with yet another type of virus—the human papilloma virus.

All of these carcinogenic viruses have one thing in common. When they infect a human cell, they bring with them new genes that in some way alter the host cell's DNA. In some instances the virus itself introduces a cancer-causing gene, called an *oncogene*, into the DNA of the host. Other viruses incorporate their DNA into that of the host in such a location that host-cell oncogenes are turned on. Whatever the method, the result is essentially the same: uncontrolled cell division—cancer.

In the 1970s a vaccine was administered to chickens that was supposed to protect them from a fatal cancer called Marek's disease. It was an avian affliction that cost poultry farmers up to $200 million a year in lost revenues in the United States alone. Interestingly and quite unexpectedly, the chickens that were inoculated not only received protection from Marek's; they also grew bigger, stronger, and healthier and laid more eggs than unvaccinated chickens. Why? The implication was that the Marek's virus was doing much more than causing cancers. Chickens believed to be healthy were, in actuality, chronically infected with Marek's virus. The infection, although subclinical and undiagnosed, was having a subtle effect on the health of the chickens.

A very intriguing hypothesis indeed, and it raised the specter of possible low-level chronic viral infections in humans. Could we be suffering from our own undiagnosed yet debilitating viruses? Many virologists today believe so. They feel that the known viral diseases that afflict humankind—and there are many—are merely the tip of the iceberg. Paul W. Ewald, of Amherst University, in his book *Plague Time*, presents the theory that heart disease, mental disorders, diabetes, and arthritis may in many instances be the result of chronic bacterial and viral infections. One's height, intelligence, and even personality might be influenced by persistent viruses that our immune system simply cannot wipe out.

What a sobering thought. Regrettably, supporting evidence, although circumstantial, has been found in the form of a very strange virus. It is called *Borna virus*, and it infects a wide range of mammals, including monkeys and humans. Once in the animal it heads straight for the brain, particularly the limbic system, that region where emotions originate. Within the nucleus of these brain cells the virus sets up a long-term persistent infection, reproducing and spreading without killing the cells.

The outcome of Borna virus infection in mammals other than humans is dramatic. Aggression, hyperactivity, depression, learning problems, and altered sexual behavior often develop. Animals display a wide range of neurotic and psychotic behaviors. And a mid-1990s study of human schizophrenics conducted by Kathryn Carbone of Johns Hopkins University and Royce W. Waldrip II at the University of Maryland found that 17 percent had Borna virus antibodies in their blood, compared to 3 percent of a nonschizophrenic control group. More recent research found traces of a retrovirus in 30 percent of patients who had recently developed schizophrenia.

Other compelling findings implicate yet another virus—a human herpesvirus known as CMV—in atherosclerosis, or hardening of the arteries. In several studies the virus has turned up in the arterial tissue of people suffering this disease. Furthermore, presence of the virus has been shown to accelerate atherosclerosis in heart transplant patients.

The presence of antibodies to a virus or even the virus itself does not unequivocally demonstrate a causal relationship between the microbe and a specific disease. Both healthy and sick people have many harmless germs residing within them. But it does give one pause. And the circumstantial evidence concerning a link between viruses and chronic diseases continues to mount. Hypertension (high blood pressure), stroke, and kidney disease, so prevalent among inner-city African-Americans, may well be brought on by infection with a virus carried by mice and rats. It is the hantavirus, a particularly virulent microbe that also causes an acute and deadly hemorrhagic fever and pulmonary disease (see Chapter 7, "Emerging Viruses").

Some viruses even play the dastardly trick of turning the body's own defenses against itself—a sort of friendly fire. The immune system, designed to fight microbial invaders, mounts an assault against its own cells instead. But why would a defense system, perfected over two billion years of evolution, go so awry? Shouldn't an army of protective cells be better able to distinguish friend from foe? Yes, it should, but remember that over the millennia viruses have been evolving and adapting along with us. These microbial masters of guerrilla warfare have devised methods of infiltrating our front lines and turning our own guns against us.

Our Immune System and Autoimmunity

The immune system is a collection of tissues and cells that vigilantly patrol the body for invading germs. Chief among these tissues and cells is an amazingly diverse array of white blood cells. They are the guts of the system. Flowing through the blood as well as the lymphatic vessels of the body, white blood cells collect in the spleen, tonsils, adenoids, appendix, small intestine, and dozens of lymph nodes. There they lie in wait for invading microorganisms with whom they do constant battle. Understanding the immune system is understanding our many different kinds of white blood cells.

Nonspecific Response

All white blood cells can be grouped broadly into several different types. The most primitive and least specialized are the *phagocytes* and *natural killer cells*. Phagocytes ooze along like so many amoebas, gobbling up bacteria and viruses they encounter along the way. They are nonspecific in their action and will eat and digest any type of germ. The *macrophage*, meaning literally "big eater," is a common phagocyte that we will encounter in later chapters.

Like phagocytes, natural killer cells are nonspecific in their immune response, but they do not attack free-roaming germs. Their targets are body cells that have gone bad—those that harbor viruses or have turned cancerous. Natural killer cells also have a mode of action different from phagocytes; they kill not by engulfing but by punching holes in the cell membrane.

Nonspecific immune responses such as these are an important line of defense. They are, in fact, the only immune system possessed by invertebrates—simple boneless animals such as insects, worms, clams, and starfish. Unfortunately, humans need much more. And they have much more—another class of white blood cells, the *lymphocytes*.

Specific Response

Without question lymphocytes handle the lion's share of defense against microbial attack. They are the infantry, the cavalry, and the air force all rolled into one. Make that two, for although all lymphocytes look alike under the microscope, there are actually two very distinct lymphocyte populations—the B lymphocytes (B cells) and the T lymphocytes (T cells).

B cells. Mature B cells pump out protein molecules called *antibodies*. It is their sole function. They do this in response to microorganisms, but only after they have come in contact with these microorganisms. And the antibodies that are produced are very specific. When a poliovirus, for example, turns on certain B cells, these cells produce antibodies that destroy only polioviruses. Measles viruses turn on different B cells that make only measles antibodies.

There are about ten trillion B cells coursing through the blood and lymphatic system of a healthy person at any given moment. This B cell population consists of a hundred million different B cells, enabling them, collectively, to recognize any type of foreign cell or particle. What they actually recognize are specific surface proteins called *antigens* (*anti*body *gen*erating). The antibodies that B cells produce in response to this recognition make up about one-fifth of the proteins found in blood. These proteins are most effective in dealing with bacteria. Viruses, on the other hand, because they reside within cells, are protected from antibody assault and must be dealt with by the other arm of the immune system—T cells.

T cells. With T cells the story of man against microbe becomes a bit more complex. For starters there are several kinds of T cells, the most important being the *helper Ts* (also called *T4s*) and the *killer Ts* (also called *T8s*). Killer and helper T cells do not respond to free bacteria, viruses, or other pathogenic agents lurking in our bodies. Unlike B cells, they cannot recognize these intruders. What they can and do recognize are our own body cells that have become infected with microorganisms. How they respond depends on whether they are killer T or helper T cells.

Killer Ts get their name because they kill. They are the only T cells that do. Their primary targets are body cells that harbor viruses. Like the bee that sacrifices itself for the greater good of the hive, cells infected with viruses serve themselves up to be slaughtered by killer T cells. In so doing, they prevent further viral multiplication and expose already existing viruses to B cells and their antibodies as well as phagocytes.

Sometimes, however, the cure is worse than the infection. Chronic sufferers of hepatitis B, for example, experience extensive liver damage even though the virus causing the disease is fairly harmless. Destruction of liver cells is a consequence not of viral activity but of killer T cell action. And in chronic fatigue syndrome, a debilitating malady that has researchers perplexed, the culprit once again seems to be an overly zealous immune system. The immune response, probably initiated by human herpesvirus 6, simply refuses to shut off, ultimately wearing down the body.

Overreaction notwithstanding, up to this point the immune system seems quite adequate and comprehensive. B cells produce antibodies that, with help from phagocytes, destroy free microbes. Killer T cells take care of any germs that might find their way into body cells. Need there be more? What possible purpose could helper T cells serve? Certainly, it may seem, not a very vital one. Even the name, *helper*, implies a subordinate role. Tell that to a dying AIDS patient, for it is primarily the helper T cells that are destroyed by HIV.

Helper T cells are the glue that holds the entire immune system together. Their secretions mobilize every other branch of the system, and they are anything but subordinate. Phagocytes, B cells, and killer Ts are all turned on by interaction with helper T cells. And when the white cells triumph over the microbial marauders and the battle has been won, it is the helper Ts that play a central role in shutting down the system.

Actually, after an infection subsides, the immune system, which has been engaged in active combat, does not shut down. It merely settles into a quiet vigil. But certain B cells and T cells, called *memory cells*, that have survived the battle remain in our bodies. These memory cells, upon encountering the same germ in the future, will immediately flood the blood-stream with antibodies and white blood cells that overwhelm the microscopic invaders. Pathogens will be thwarted before ever gaining a foothold. And therein lies the phenomenon of long-lasting immunity after recovery from an infection. Vaccination induces this immunity by introducing dead or weakened germs into the body. Conferring immunity, through its memory cells, is a fundamental and vital property of the immune system.

So fine-tuned is this system of defense that one marvels at how homeless microbes could possibly carve out a niche for themselves inside the human body. Yet they do, and with alarming regularity. One ingenious method they employ is called *molecular mimicry*. Make the surface of the virus similar enough to a nerve or muscle cell, and the T and B white blood cells will not recognize it as a foreign invader. Disguised in this way, microbes will not be attacked. They will be tolerated by the immune system. But they are wolves in lambs' clothing.

Aside from the obvious problem of allowing germs free access to body cells, molecular mimicry causes additional trouble. The similarity of germs to certain body cells in some instances triggers an immune assault on those body cells. Because the attack is on "self" tissues, the resulting disorder is termed *autoimmune disease*. When insulin-producing cells of the pancreas are targeted, the result is juvenile diabetes. In rheumatoid arthritis it is the cartilage and lubricating tissues of the joints that are literally eaten away by immune system cells. Multiple sclerosis sufferers are victims of yet another kind of autoimmune attack, this time on cells of the central nervous system.

Origin of Viruses

It appears that somehow, some way, viruses will find a means to gain biological profit at our expense. As the historical record shows, they have been doing so for thousands of years. The pockmarked mummified face of Ramses V is mute testimony to the presence of smallpox in ancient Egypt. Bas-relief hieroglyphics from that period also depict a priest with shriveled legs, suggestive of polio. And without question viral infection predates ancient Egypt. Almost certainly the earliest cave dwellers had viruses to contend with. The ways in which viruses slip into cells and seize control could only come about through a very long association in which viruses have adapted and are continually adapting to their hosts.

Exactly when the association began is still a matter of conjecture. One theory proposes that viruses, because they are simpler than cells, actually arrived on the scene first. According to this hypothesis, nucleic acids increased in complexity until they became the stuff of cells. Along the way, simpler DNA and RNA strands were left behind to learn the ways of parasitism—to become the stuff of viruses.

Although once popular, this theory is now considered unlikely. A more probable scenario is that viruses have evolved from bits of cellular genetic material that escaped from their cells aeons ago. Over time, according to the "escaped gene" hypothesis, these scraps of host-derived nucleic acid developed the ability to be independent, self-replicating, intracellular parasites. They became viruses.

One scientist, the noted British astronomer Fred Hoyle, has even proposed that viruses originally fell, and continue to fall, from outer space. Not exactly a consensus among today's virologists. Whatever their origin, once viruses established themselves on this planet they were a force to be reckoned with. And remarkably, it was not as agents of disease that they may have exerted their most profound effects. It was as agents of evolutionary change.

Viruses as Agents of Genetic Change

The first insight that viruses may do much more than make us sick came from studies with Rous sarcoma virus in the 1970s. The virus causes a deadly cancer in chickens. It does so by inserting a cancer-causing gene, an oncogene, right into the DNA of the host cell—a process called *integration.*

Scientists were curious about this oncogene and began taking a closer look at it. To their astonishment, it turned out to be a very common gene found routinely in healthy chickens. Apparently the sarcoma virus was snatching the gene from the host cell and carrying it off to other cells in other chickens. During the abduction, close association with viral genes altered the normal chicken gene, turning it into a cancer inducer.

Stranger still, this kidnapped gene was incredibly ubiquitous, appearing in a wide range of vertebrates, including fish, mice, cows, and even humans. Perhaps this ubiquity was not coincidental. Perhaps viruses were disseminating the gene not only to other chickens but throughout the animal kingdom. Taken to its logical conclusion, viruses could be agents of dispersal for a whole host of genes. This would rank the virus right up there with sexual reproduction as a major force in bringing about genetic variability and ultimately the evolution of species.

Then in 1977 a scientific discovery was made that truly stunned the genetics community. In that year scientists stumbled on *introns* in the genes of chickens and rabbits. An intron is a stretch of meaningless DNA—DNA that codes for no proteins and has, as yet, no discernible function. Not surprisingly, scientists refer to it as *junk DNA.*

Further investigations have turned up introns in many other animals, including humans. In fact the more highly evolved an organism, the more meaningless DNA it seems to possess. Amazingly, more than 95 percent of our own DNA is worthless stretches of introns.

Could this junk DNA be leftover bits and pieces of ancient viral infections, a fossil legacy of our evolutionary past? Could the vast majority of our genetic material be useless scraps of invisible germs that have crept into our chromosomes over the aeons? Yes, indeed, it could. Since the discovery of junk DNA, studies by molecular biologists have demonstrated that certain stretches of human DNA look remarkably like the genomes of certain viruses. And some viral DNA found in humans is identical to bits found in our closest nonhuman relatives, the chimpanzees. Researchers hypothesize that ten million or fifty million years ago this virus slipped into the DNA of a primate that would later evolve into chimpanzees and humans. It might even have been a virus that at the time caused a deadly epidemic—a prehistoric AIDS. Now it is merely excess baggage in the descendant cells of those that survived its terror, a silent reminder of some ancient viral infection, a guest that came to dinner and simply would not leave.

Beyond the Virus—the Prion

Molecular biology is much like Alice's Wonderland; things just keep getting curiouser and curiouser. First to be discovered was the bacterium, a tiny one-celled organism that grew inside us and made us sick. Then came the virus, an even tinier particle that actually entered our cells and became part of them. It also made us sick. Strangest and most remarkable of all, however, is an infectious particle isolated and identified in 1982. Not a living cell, not even a virus, the tiny particle baffled scientists because it appeared to be pure protein. There was a total absence of genetic material, which would rule out the ability to reproduce, and yet it was undoubtedly infectious, causing a number of fatal diseases that literally punched holes in the brain.

As it turned out, the particles, given the name *prions* for "proteinaceous infectious particles," do not replicate. What they do, however, is just as deadly. When prions come in contact with certain normal host cell proteins, they cause those proteins to flip into a distorted shape that resembles the prion. In what appears to be a chain reaction of sorts, these newly deformed proteins then convert other neighboring normal proteins. Enzymes that usually break down brain proteins when they are no longer needed cannot act upon these abnormal molecules. When enough normal protein has been altered, disease results. Fascinating stuff, this molecular biology.

Kuru is one of only a few known prion diseases. It affected natives of Papua New Guinea, who contracted it when family members ate the brains of recently deceased loved ones. It was a customary show of respect that has since been discontinued.

The prion also causes a rare neurological disorder called Creutzfeldt-Jakob disease (CJD). The famed choreographer George Balanchine died of CJD. It is among animals, however, that the prion is most devastating, causing, in cattle, the neurological ailment *mad cow disease*. The disorder was discovered in 1984 when a veterinarian was called to a farm in southern England, where a dairy cow was displaying unusual behavior—panic, aggression, and a staggering gait. By 1985 more cows began exhibiting signs of the mysterious malady. The disease was invariably fatal, and examination of dead cows' brains showed them to be riddled with holes, like so much Swiss cheese. *Bovine spongiform encephalopathy* (BSE), the medically correct name for mad cow disease, had claimed its first victims. But an epidemic was brewing in England, and by 1992 through 1993 almost one thousand new cases were appearing weekly. Then the disease began to wane. Nonetheless, as of July 2000 more than 176,000 cows had succumbed to the prion-caused infection in Great Britain. Scattered cases also appeared in eighteen other European countries, Canada, and Japan. The vast majority, however—better than 99 percent—were confined to the United Kingdom. Mad cows and Englishmen.

But from where had this disease come, a disease unknown until 1984? By the late 1980s epidemiologists and infectious disease specialists began piecing together the "mad cow" puzzle. Cattle are routinely fed discarded animal parts—meat and bone—which have been ground up and added to the feed. This meat-and-bone meal provides cheap protein, necessary for proper milk production. Unfortunately, some cattle were fed remnants from sheep infected with scrapie, a brain-wasting disorder known since the 1700s that is similar to mad cow and caused by the same infectious agent. Before 1981, the carcasses of ruminants (cows, sheep, goats) were subjected to high heat and use of organic solvents to remove fat before being processed into feed. This had been sufficient to destroy any contaminating prions. But changes in the rendering process, done for economic reasons, reduced the heat and eliminated the organic solvent, allowing the as-yet-undiscovered prions to escape inactivation.

To remedy the situation, Britain destroyed millions of animals as a precautionary measure and instituted strict laws banning the use of ruminant body parts as sources of protein in cattle feed. In the United States, there have been no reported cases of mad cows, and to ensure that America stays

BSE-free, laws were passed in 1989 prohibiting importation of live ruminants from countries where BSE was known to exist. By 1997 it was expanded to include ruminant products such as meat, meat-and-bone meal, and offal from all of Europe.

With significant numbers of cattle being infected, the question arose as to whether a health risk existed if meat from these sick cows entered the food supply. Initially experts believed it "most unlikely that BSE will have any implications for human health" (*Secret Agents: The Menace of Emerging Infections,* by Madeline Drexler). They were wrong. In 1996, ten cases of a new form of Creutzfeldt-Jakob disease surfaced in the United Kingdom, featuring bizarre behavioral and personality changes, staggering, and dementia. And it appeared in startlingly young patients, averaging twenty-eight years of age. The prion had made the cross-species jump from ruminants to humans. To date there is no cure for the disease, which is invariable fatal.

There is also no quick and easy way to check for prion infection in cows. The presence of the BSE agent in tissue is generally determined by injecting mice with material believed to be infected and observing the mouse. These mouse inoculation studies can take nearly two years. Special staining procedures can also be used to detect abnormal prion protein in tissues, but the tests are often inaccurate and inconclusive.

Thankfully, the few known prion diseases are all quite rare. Even the variant CJD, linked to the ingestion of mad cow beef, has resulted in less than two hundred cases worldwide since 1996. And although the incubation period is long—ten years or more—and many more cases will be presenting over the next decade, it is still the viruses and bacteria that pose the greatest menace to humankind—a menace that is only now being fully realized, with the emergence of new and incredibly deadly viral infections and increasingly drug-resistant bacteria.

The Gathering Storm—Emerging Viruses

The twentieth century has witnessed the eradication of one of the worst viral afflictions ever to plague humanity—smallpox. By the year 2005 polio will hopefully have suffered a similar fate. Add to that the successes antibiotics have enjoyed on the bacterial front, and it is small wonder that microbiologists were lulled into a false sense of security. In 1969 the U.S. surgeon general, William H. Stewart, declared that "the war against infectious disease had been won." Students of biology were steered away from the study of pathogenicity because it was believed that all the important work had already been done.

Then came AIDS . . . and Ebola and Lassa fever and Marburg and dengue fever and West Nile virus. They came, for the most part, from the steamy jungles of the world. Lush tropical rain forests are ablaze with deadly viruses. And changing lifestyles as well as changing environmental conditions are flushing them out. Air travel, deforestation, and global warming are forcing never-before-encountered viruses to suddenly cross the path of humanity. The result—emerging viruses.

Today roughly five thousand vials of exotic viruses sit, freeze-dried, at Yale University—imports from the rain forests. They await the outbreak of diseases that can be ascribed to them. Many are carried by insects and are termed *arboviruses* (*ar*thropod *bor*ne). Others, of even greater concern, are airborne and can simply be breathed in. Some, no doubt, could threaten humanity's very existence. Joshua Lederberg, 1958 winner of the Nobel Prize in Physiology or Medicine and foremost authority on emerging viruses, warned in a December 1990 article in *Discover* magazine, "It is still not comprehended widely that AIDS is a natural, almost predictable phenomenon. It is not going to be a unique event. Pandemics are not acts of God, but are built into the ecological relations between viruses, animal species, and human species. . . . There will be more surprises, because our fertile imagination does not begin to match all the tricks that nature can play." According to Lederberg, "The survival of humanity is not preordained. . . . The single biggest threat to man's continued dominance on the planet is the virus" (*A Dancing Matrix*, by Robin Marantz Henig).

7

Emerging Viruses

Sickness comes on horseback, but goes away on foot.

—W. C. HAZLITT

IN 1969 MICHAEL CRICHTON wrote a terrifying book called *The Androm-
eda Strain*. It chronicled events surrounding the emergence of a virus so
deadly that it could have wiped out humanity. The book was science fiction.

In 1994 Richard Preston wrote a terrifying book called *The Hot Zone*.
It chronicled events surrounding the emergence of viruses so deadly that
they could have wiped out humanity. The book was science fact, an account
of two viruses named after their places of discovery—*Marburg* (a city in
Germany) and *Ebola* (a river in Zaire).

Marburg

On a hot August day in 1967 three factory workers for the vaccine-
producing company Behring Works developed muscle aches and mild
fevers. Possibly some sort of flu, doctors first thought. As the days dragged
on, however, it became apparent that this was no flu. The workers became
nauseated and began to vomit. Diarrhea set in. At the same time their eyes

became severely bloodshot and they developed a painful red rash—the result of blood clotting in the thousands of capillaries just under the skin. Their throats became so raw that they could not swallow and had to be fed intravenously. But the virus was just warming up. Within ten days of the onset of symptoms they began vomiting and defecating blood.

Marburg, Ebola, and several other devastating viral infections are termed *hemorrhagic fevers* because sufferers start bleeding profusely in the latter stages of the disease. With the body's clotting factors exhausted, blood pours out of every orifice, taking sloughed-off body tissues with it. In an agony of crimson gore the victim "crashes and bleeds out" to use the expression of doctors familiar with the disease. Blood and Marburg viruses gush in all directions. If the virus lands on another human, the horrid cycle of infection will begin again.

In total, thirty-one Europeans were infected with Marburg, including six people in Frankfurt, Germany, and a veterinarian and his wife in Yugoslavia. Seven died. Then Marburg vanished just as suddenly as it had appeared.

In the aftermath of the onslaught scientists worked frantically to answer the most basic questions. What kind of virus was it? Where had it come from? To answer the second question first, it was discovered early on that all of the people who originally became ill were handling monkeys or monkey tissues. Furthermore, all of the monkeys were African green monkeys imported from Uganda in three separate shipments. Wild monkeys are routinely imported from Africa and Asia by research facilities throughout the world. Manufacturers of polio vaccine use monkeys to develop their product since poliovirus will grow well in monkey kidney cells. Each year about ten thousand of them make it to the United States. Obviously something was wrong with the batch that went to Germany in 1967.

As it turned out, almost half of the monkeys first shipped from Uganda were dead on arrival. Not surprisingly, many had died of massive hemorrhages. Whatever was killing the monkeys back in their jungle homes had been imported to Europe and was jumping to a new species—humans. The virus was *emerging*.

When a virus jumps to a new animal species it, as a rule, is uncommonly deadly. The new host has never been exposed to the virus, and a relationship based on coevolution has not developed. For this reason scientists did not believe the green monkey to be Marburg's natural host. The virus was even more devastating to these primates than to humans, killing with a ferocity approaching 100 percent. Most likely there was a reservoir of Marburg viruses hiding in some other, as yet unknown, rain forest animal.

Over the next few years the WHO as well as the United States and Europe sent teams of scientists to Kenya and Uganda to scour the countryside in search of that animal. They caught and tested tens of thousands of monkeys, apes, rodents, mosquitoes, ticks, bats, and cats. Unfortunately, the animal in which the Marburg virus resided naturally and harmlessly proved very elusive, and no reservoir for the virus was ever found.

Electron micrographs of blood and tissue samples from Marburg victims did reveal that, wherever its hiding place, the virus was unlike any other. Whereas most viruses are spherical or of similar shape, Marburg looked like a short piece of yarn. When it "amplified" itself within a cell, producing thousands of viral copies, it resembled a bowl of entangled spaghetti. Hence the agent of Marburg hemorrhagic fever was dubbed a *filovirus*, *filo* being Latin for "thread." No other virus looked like Marburg.

Since the 1967 German outbreak the virus has struck again only twice, in 1976 and again in 1990. Four people in all were infected, all Europeans, and all contracted the disease during travels in Africa. One person died. Today the virus sits, freeze-dried, in just a few laboratories throughout the world.

The scientific community is not actively engaged in studying Marburg because it is so "hot." A hot virus is one that spreads easily, kills quickly, with a high mortality rate, and has no cure or preventive vaccine. The hottest viruses, of which Marburg is a charter member, require very special handling. Doctors must wear cumbersome "space suits" with independent air supplies to keep all parts of their bodies from direct contact with the pathogen. Additional rubber gloves are worn beneath the suit and sometimes even over the suit, as further protection against accidental cuts or punctures while working with scalpels and hypodermic needles. Animals and tissue specimens are often handled in sealed, airtight glass and steel boxes with permanently attached gloves. The name of the game is viral containment.

To denote the level of precaution necessary in dealing with such a contagious killer, the army refers to a hot virus as a *Biosafety Level 4 (BL 4) agent*. A Level 4 laboratory is kept under constant negative air pressure—

a pressure lower than its surroundings. This ensures that the flow of air—always into the room—will prevent escape of airborne viruses. The United States Army Medical Research Institute of Infectious Diseases (USAM-RIID) operates a BL 4 lab at Fort Detrick, just outside Washington, D.C. A similar laboratory exists at the CDC in Atlanta, Georgia. It was, in fact, the emergence of the Marburg virus that prompted construction of a maximum containment facility at the CDC.

When leaving a Level 4 lab, scientists must be decontaminated. They must be bathed in ultraviolet light, a radiation that chops up the virus's genetic material. They must undergo a seven-minute chemical shower, one that no opportunistic microbe can survive.

By comparison, HIV is only a Level 2 virus. No special suits, air pressures, or decontamination (decon) procedures are required. This is because the disease it causes, AIDS, although more lethal than Marburg, is not easily contracted. HIV is a very fragile virus and one that is not spread through casual contact. It dies within seconds of exposure to air and cannot be transmitted through the air. Scientists believe Marburg can.

Marburg killed about 25 percent of the people it infected, making it an extremely lethal virus. Many of humanity's worst plagues did not have mortality figures that high. Yellow fever, for example, a deadly viral disease transmitted by the bite of a female mosquito (male mosquitoes do not bite), usually killed only one in ten. Yet Marburg was not the worst of the hemorrhagic fevers to come out of the jungles of Africa. Nine years after the emergence of Marburg, in the central African nations of Sudan and Zaire, an even deadlier virus struck. It came to be known as *Ebola*.

Ebola

Ebola first introduced itself to humanity in the southern Sudan in July 1976. A quiet, unassuming man named Mr. Yu. G. became ill and died an agonizing and bloody death. From him the virus radiated outward, infecting friends, mistresses, and family members. Before the outbreak ran its course, 284 people became infected and 150 died, a death rate of just over 50 percent.

Then, in September of that year, Ebola struck again, this time in Zaire. Ebola Zaire turned out to be a slightly different strain from Ebola Sudan;

it was a super-Ebola that killed a staggering 90 percent of its victims. For several months late in 1976 it swept through fifty villages, killing 325 of the 358 people it infected.

The way it killed was not pretty. The Ebola virus can attack and amplify itself in virtually any body tissue except bone and perhaps skeletal muscle. First come the searing headaches, fever, and muscle pain. Then the bleeding starts. When internal hemorrhaging first occurs, the body's clotting factors are called into play. Organs such as the liver and spleen are transformed into hardened, desiccated masses of coagulated blood and tissue. The kidneys, filtering organs for the body, become so clogged with clumped blood that they cease to function. A tremendous burden is placed on the heart as it attempts to pump this congealing mess through thousands of miles of blood vessels. When all the clotting factor available has been depleted, uncontrolled bleeding commences. The virus is now running amok, amplifying itself by the billions as it destroys the body. Capillaries deteriorate, and blood flows into the lungs, stomach, and intestine. The skin may balloon as blood leaks into the underlying tissue. Victims weep blood. Ebola is transforming its host's innards into viral soup. Mercifully death soon follows, often from shock (due to blood loss and lowered blood pressure), heart failure, or lung congestion.

The Ebola viruses proved to be close cousins of Marburg. All were filoviruses that, under the probing beam of the electron microscope, appeared nearly identical. All had similar genetic material—a single strand of RNA. And like Marburg, no natural host was ever found for either strain of Ebola. To this day we have no idea where in the rain forests of Africa this serial killer lurks.

Just as with the Marburg scare, the Ebola outbreaks in Africa ended as quickly as they began. Like a hurricane ripping through the countryside, destroying those homes less able to withstand its onslaught, Ebola ravaged those unfortunate enough to cross its path. And then it was gone. The hemorrhagic fever would reemerge, however, in May of 1995 and then again in the year 2000. Before its monthlong bloody rampage was over, 203 Zaireans would die a horrific death in the 1995 outbreak. Almost as many Ugandans would perish at the turn of the millennium.

Undoubtedly we have not seen the last of Ebola. But why, if it was so lethal to humans, did it not destroy millions, as epidemics of smallpox, influenza, and the Black Death had done? Perhaps it was too deadly for its own good. As Richard Preston points out in *The Hot Zone*, "Ebola does in ten days what it takes AIDS ten years to do." In ten years HIV has much greater opportunity to transmit itself to other humans than Ebola does in ten days.

Even more significant, the filoviruses are apparently not as contagious as originally feared. Although Marburg and Ebola can infect and kill monkeys that inhale the virus, airborne transmission is not easily accomplished. And transmission from human to human through casual contact is even less likely. During the outbreaks of 1976, the spread of Ebola was not the result of people greeting one another in the street or frequenting the same restaurants. Ironically, it was the hospitals that were largely responsible for the miniepidemics. Many hospitals were little more than beat-up shacks run by Christian missionaries. Medical supplies were almost nonexistent. When patients came in for antimalarial medication or treatment for various and sundry ailments, the same needles were used over and over again, with little more than a quick rinse between injections. Small wonder hospitals became nothing more than death camps, with nuns unwittingly injecting lethal viruses into healthy people.

In 1989 Ebola even made its way to the United States, winding up at the Hazelton Research Products facility in Reston, Virginia. Not surprisingly, it arrived through the importation of research monkeys, five hundred of them. The monkeys, however, were not from Africa, and they were not green monkeys. This particular Ebola strain had come from the Philippines. When the monkeys started dying and a filovirus was found in their blood, medical experts went into a panic. USAMRIID and the CDC were called in. All of the surviving monkeys were destroyed, and the entire Hazelton facility was scrubbed with bleach and deconned with formaldehyde gas. Thankfully Ebola Reston proved nonpathogenic to humans. No one died. No one even got sick. But several workers did test positive for Ebola antibodies in their blood. They had been infected. America had dodged a viral bullet.

It is interesting to note that, during one of the Ebola outbreaks in Africa, the blood of one nun, a survivor of the disease, was repeatedly tapped for its Ebola antibodies. When injected into a person during the early stages of Ebola fever, it sometimes proved beneficial. Recently researchers have taken this antibody therapy and run with it, producing certain of these immune system molecules that will bind specifically to proteins on the surface of Ebola-infected cells. When administered to mice twenty-four hours before infection with Ebola, they were able to ward off infection. Some mice even received protection when treatment was given *after* Ebola exposure. Although not a vaccine, antibody therapy, if it proves successful in human trials, can offer short-term postexposure prophylaxis.

Filoviruses are not the only pathogens emerging from the rain forests. Nor are they the only Level 4 viruses making headlines. Other deadly viruses exist that may, because of their infectivity and modes of transmission, pose even greater threats to humankind. Lassa fever, dengue fever, and Korean hemorrhagic fever are all caused by hot viruses that merit close monitoring. All have caused fatalities in the United States.

Lassa

Lassa fever is a hemorrhagic disease endemic to western Africa, where it is responsible for about five thousand deaths a year. It is a brutal killer in the fashion of Marburg or Ebola. Science first became aware of Lassa in 1969, when it struck down American nurses in a church-run hospital in Nigeria. The symptoms of the disease—high fever, throat ulcers, and severe hemorrhaging—were scarily reminiscent of Marburg, which had been discovered two years earlier. Under the electron microscope, however, Lassa virus was spherical, looking nothing like a filovirus. And when the new pathogen was mixed with Marburg antibodies, no reaction occurred. Lassa was stimulating the body to produce antibodies different from Marburg. They were entirely different viruses.

Not only did Lassa not react with Marburg antibodies; it did not react with any known antibodies. This could mean only one thing: the medical establishment had yet another hot virus on its hands.

Once again the hunt was on for the source, or natural host, of the virus. A gut feeling told researchers that it was not an arbovirus. For one thing, all cases appeared to have occurred indoors. For another, the disease attacked primarily adults. As a rule, insect-carried diseases show a preference for children because they play in the wet breeding grounds of mosquitoes, mites, ticks, etc.

The hunch proved correct. More than 640 animals, mostly small mammals such as mice, rats, and bats, were captured in and around the affected villages. Blood was collected. Lungs, hearts, spleens, and kidneys were surgically removed. All specimens were placed in liquid nitrogen and shipped overseas to the Special Pathogens Branch of the CDC for testing. When the results came in, one animal turned up positive for Lassa virus—*Mastomys matalensis*, a common brown rat.

The Black Death and typhus were both monstrous killers, stealthily introduced into human communities by the rat. But these diseases were actually transmitted to humans by fleas or lice living on and biting the diseased rodents. Was this the mode of transmission for Lassa, or did the rats themselves bite human victims? Lassa sufferers did not recall being bitten. But one researcher was urinated on by an angry rat as he held it. Two weeks later the scientist died of Lassa fever.

As it turned out, the urine of infected rats was teeming with viruses. And the animals were ubiquitous throughout eight countries in western Africa, finding human dwellings particularly to their liking. They urinated on food, floors, bedding, and even people as they slept. The tiniest break in the skin would afford the virus a portal into a human host.

Lassa virus, like Marburg and Ebola, has made brief excursions out of its native land. In 1989 a man in Chicago died of the disease. He had contracted it while visiting his mother in Africa, who also lay dying of Lassa. But no one caught the disease from him. Yet another viral-emergence scare went by the boards.

Emergence outside Africa never happened because Lassa is not very adept at hopping from one human to another. Mercifully, most hot viruses are not. But what if a Lassa-carrying rat had made its way into an airplane headed for Chicago? What if the rat was able to infect American rats after it disembarked? That may have happened—not for Lassa, but for another rodent-borne hot virus, the hantavirus.

Hantavirus

In the 1950s the United States was part of a United Nations contingent fighting a war in Korea. Battle casualties ran high. But unbeknownst to the army, some two thousand of its fighting men were engaged in another battle, with a strange and deadly virus. Several hundred lost that battle. The disease they succumbed to came to be called *Korean hemorrhagic fever*. Following the GI deaths a massive effort was made to isolate the microbe responsible for Korean hemorrhagic fever—more recently renamed *hemorrhagic fever with renal syndrome*. The task proved very daunting, however, and it was not until 1976—twenty-odd years later—that the offending virus was found. It was given the name *Hantaan* in honor of a nearby river in Korea.

The Hantaan virus (subsequently shortened to *hantavirus*) was first discovered in the lung tissue of its natural host, the striped field mouse, in which it caused no illness. But different strains would soon be found in different rodents as well. In Seoul, Korea's densely populated capital, the vector was a common inner-city rat. It carried a hantavirus that produced typical, though less severe, symptoms of fever, internal bleeding, and kidney failure in humans. Kidney involvement seemed to be a hallmark of the disease.

The implication of hanta-carrying rodents in Seoul were scary. By the early 1980s Korea had become a major exporter of goods to the United States. What if one Korean import was not an article of clothing but a stowaway rat—a hantavirus-infected rat?

With that thought in mind, army and CDC scientists combed the harbors of port cities such as Baltimore, Philadelphia, New Orleans, New York, and San Francisco, searching for rats. When the rats were tested, Seoul hantavirus turned up virtually everywhere. Scientists were puzzled. If the hantavirus was so prevalent, why weren't more people sick? Actually they were, but not the explosive, rapid-death kind of sick. The American-variety hantavirus was a more silent killer, taking its toll while going unnoticed—until the late 1980s, when studies at Johns Hopkins confirmed hantavirus in cases of hypertension and chronic kidney failure at a frequency five times greater than in the general population. No small discovery when one considers that thirty-five million people in the United States suffer and die prematurely from high blood pressure.

There was also an exception to the nonexplosive killing habits of the virus. A hot hantavirus struck the midwestern United States in 1993 like a bombshell.

It all began on Friday, May 14, in the Four Corners area of New Mexico (where the boundaries of New Mexico, Arizona, Colorado, and Utah intersect). A Navajo Indian, young and athletic, suddenly began gasping for breath while driving to his fiancée's funeral. He was rushed to the hospital but died later that day. His bride-to-be had passed away five days earlier. Both experienced mild flulike symptoms before suffering severe respiratory distress.

Over the next few weeks a dozen more cases were reported and the CDC was called in. What most alarmed doctors was how rapidly the disease killed. According to Denise Grady in her 1993 *Discover* article, "Death in the Corners," "One patient who sat up in bed in the morning talking and eating breakfast was on a respirator by the afternoon and was dead that night."

The CDC felt that whatever it was dealing with, it certainly was hot and decided that blood and tissue samples of the dead should be examined in its BL 4 facility. Autopsies performed on the victims revealed severe pulmonary edema. The fluid of the blood had leaked out of capillaries and into the lungs' air sacs. Seepage was so great that the lungs had swelled to more than twice their normal weight. Deaths were literally the result of drowning.

What could have produced such extraordinary symptoms? Research focused on about two dozen infectious diseases, including influenza, plague, and anthrax as well as the hot hemorrhagics Ebola, Marburg, and Lassa. The procedure was quite straightforward. Antibodies against the germs were much easier to detect in the blood than the actual microorganisms, especially if they were viral. So scientists took blood from the victims, separated out the antibody-containing serum, and mixed it with different known germs. If a reaction occurred, then the person had to have been infected with that particular microbe. Sometimes, in lieu of the germ itself, a bit of its surface protein was used.

By early June 1993, barely three weeks after the initial case, the CDC had its microbe. In all the tests only one antigen reacted positively with the victims' antibodies. It was from a hantavirus. This surprised researchers. The deadliest hantavirus of Asia had caused obvious hemorrhaging, but the Four Corners hantavirus did not. And in the deadly American strain there was much more lung involvement. The disease came to be called *hantavirus pulmonary syndrome* (HPS).

Being a hantavirus, its natural host/vector was most likely a rodent. Capturing and testing of animals began. Sure enough, a mouse, the large-eared, white-bellied deer mouse, turned out to be the culprit.

But deer mice had been omnipresent in the Four Corners area for quite some time. Why were they suddenly spreading a deadly virus to people? Hantavirus lived harmlessly in the rodents, suggesting that it was not a new arrival on the scene. Had recent mutations in the genes of the hantavirus suddenly turned them lethal to humans? (Mutations are changes in the genetic material of a cell or virus that occur when it replicates.) Certainly mutation was a distinct possibility, especially since hanta was an RNA virus. RNA mutates much more readily than DNA. It is the reason scientists have identified more than seventy different hantavirus strains, carried by sixty-three different species of birds and small mammals.

Scientists were hesitant, however, to place blame on a new strain. Other environmental factors seemed even more likely to have caused the outbreak. Record snowfalls and rainfalls the previous year had produced bumper crops of the nuts, berries, and seeds—especially piñon nuts—on which rodents feed. This caused a dramatic, nearly tenfold increase in the deer mouse population. Parts of New Mexico had more than six thousand deer mice per square acre. They overran their natural habitats and invaded human dwellings, spreading the disease when viruses in their urine became airborne.

Once the method of transmission had been determined, people in the area were advised to set out traps and poison to kill any adventuresome deer mice. The strategy worked, and another national catastrophe was averted. All told, about forty hantavirus cases were reported and confirmed from the Four Corners outbreak. Twenty-five resulted in death. But deer mice are a ubiquitous American rodent, and by 2001 nearly three hundred cases of HPS had been reported in thirty-one states, with a mortality approaching 40 percent.

To date, there is no cure or licensed vaccine for hantavirus. Army scientists have, however, developed an experimental vaccine against certain of its strains—a genetically engineered product, prepared by inserting hantavirus genes into vaccinia, the tried-and-true cowpox virus. Early tests show that the vaccine is eliciting antibody production against hantavirus, a very encouraging sign.

Dengue

Dengue hemorrhagic fever (pronounced "den-gee") is the more severe form of a related disease called simply *dengue fever*. Both cause excruciating bone and joint pain from which the disease derives its common names, *breakbone fever* and *devil's crunch*. In the hemorrhagic dengue, however, internal bleeding and subsequent shock lead to death 20 percent of the time. Many experts feel dengue is the disease most likely to emerge and become America's next plague. Why?

Like its close cousin yellow fever, dengue is an arbovirus. It is spread by the bite of an arthropod. Both diseases, in fact, are transmitted by the same vector, a mosquito called *A. aegypti*. Mosquitoes are among the most efficient transmitters of disease. In Zaire it was reused hypodermic needles that spread Ebola so rapidly throughout hospitals. Well, a female mosquito (remember that only females bite) is a flying hypodermic needle. The needle, a long proboscis, is used to secure a blood meal. But before sticking her victim the mosquito goes through an odd ritual. She primes the targeted patch of skin by first spitting on it. The saliva, in addition to containing an anticoagulant that keeps the blood flowing, may be loaded with virus particles. Then Ms. *aegypti* inserts her proboscis and gorges herself on a huge quantity of blood, ballooning to four times her original weight.

At this point the mosquito becomes more than a hypodermic syringe. If the blood she ingests happens to contain dengue viruses, they will replicate themselves in her salivary glands. When she again spits and bites, woe to the hapless victim.

Now imagine tens of millions of these viral-amplifying airborne microneedles flying throughout much of Asia, Africa, and South and Central America. This is where *A. aegypti* is endemic. The mosquito thrives wherever there is standing water and winters that do not produce frost. Small wonder an estimated fifty million people worldwide are infected with dengue every year. Thankfully the vast majority contract the milder nonhemorrhagic form and usually recover completely in ten days. But instead of inducing immunity to hemorrhagic dengue, the infection does the opposite, sensitizing people and making them more prone to attack by the deadlier dengue virus. In 1981 hemorrhagic dengue was the leading cause of pediatric hospitalization in Southeast Asia. Since then there have been major outbreaks in Cuba and South America. Between January and October 1998, Brazil alone reported 475,000 cases of dengue.

Surely, you might say, tropical arboviruses do not threaten to emerge in North America. Wrong. In 1985 a ship from Japan sailed into a Texas port. Its cargo was hundreds of thousands of used tires scheduled for recapping. The tires were wet, many filled with puddles of stagnant rainwater. In that water were the larvae of a new import to America's shores—the Asian tiger mosquito, so named because of its yellow-and-black striped coloration. But it also had the temperament of a tiger, biting ferociously and with a ravenous appetite.

Each bite could be deadly, for the tiger mosquito carried dengue and a dozen or so other dangerous viruses. More important, it proved to be extremely hardy, establishing itself in seventeen southern states within a few years. By 1994 a total of 2,248 suspected cases of imported dengue were confirmed in the United States. Today it continues to expand its range and shows no signs of slowing down. Able to withstand cold winters, the tiger mosquito has already made its way at least as far north as Illinois. Global warming will only exacerbate the situation. Health officials feel it is only a matter of time before dengue, or some other arbovirus, emerges (or yellow fever reappears) from these aggressive vectors, and they are scared to death.

Although there is currently no vaccine for dengue, progress is being made. Part of the problem is that four different viruses exist, all of which cause dengue. Within a few years a vaccine may become available. In the meantime, we must fight dengue by fighting its mosquito vector, and denying it the wet breeding grounds it requires.

West Nile Virus

On August 23, 1999, a phone rang at the Bureau of Communicable Diseases in the New York City Department of Health. It was Deborah Asnis, an infectious disease specialist, calling from Flushing Hospital Medical Center in Queens, New York. She had two cases that troubled her. Both came in confused and feverish, and subsequently became so weak that they could not move their arms or legs. Several days later two more patients, an elderly man and woman, were added to the list of those being admitted with these mysterious paralysis symptoms. What strange illness was afoot?

Initial tests suggested a form of encephalitis. When serum and tissues of the victims were screened for antibodies against viruses known to cause brain inflammation, the samples came back positive for St. Louis encephalitis.

At about the same time, the Bronx Zoo began experiencing a sudden die-off of its birds. Crows seemed hardest hit. Avian autopsies showed extensive brain inflammation and hemorrhaging—acute meningoencephalitis. Could the two outbreaks be related? An answer would come through comparison of the viral DNAs found in the birds with genetic sequences of known viruses. The results were shocking to say the least. The causative agent in both bird and human infections was West Nile virus.

First discovered in the blood of a fever-ridden woman in the West Nile district of Uganda in 1937, the virus has been tracked in Africa, the Middle East, and western Asia. Before 1999, however, it had never appeared in the United States—never appeared, for that matter, in any of the Americas. West Nile belongs to the same family of viruses as those causing yellow fever and dengue. And like them, it is an arbovirus, transmitted through the bite of *Culex pipiens*, a drab, brown bloodsucker commonly known as the northern house mosquito.

There are 540 known arboviruses, 110 of them capable of causing human disease. Many are zoonotic infections, crossing over from animals that are the virus's natural reservoir to human hosts via the bite of an insect vector. Some arboviruses have an affinity for the brain and its meninges, resulting in the inflammation of encephalitis.

How did an insect-transmitted illness make it halfway around the globe to hapless victims in New York? In any one of a number of ways. A sick bird imported from an endemic region of the world; an infected mosquito stowing away on a transoceanic air flight; a human returning home from a visit to family in a developing nation. Any and/or all of these events could trigger emergence of a deadly epidemic. It was even speculated that West Nile was an act of bioterror. In April 1999 a London tabloid ran an article in which an Iraqi defector boasted the creation of a West Nile virus by Saddam Hussein "capable of destroying 97% of all life in an urban environment" (*Secret Agents: The Menace of Emerging Infections*, by Madeline Drexler). Since then, genetic sequencing of the New York strain has ruled out such a possibility. It showed that the American import could only have descended from a 1998 Israeli strain by natural mutation.

In 1999, sixty-two people were hospitalized by West Nile virus. Seven died. But the drawing of blood from New Yorkers showed thousands testing positive for antibodies to the pathogen. Obviously it silently infected many, with most experiencing no symptoms or a mild flulike course of fever, headache, and malaise before fully recovering. The figures indicate that perhaps one in a hundred infected will come down with encephalitis, with one in a thousand succumbing. Thankfully, Ebola it is not.

In the grip of such an emerging threat, New York and other municipalities sprang into immediate action. Wherever possible, areas of standing, stagnant waters—the breeding ground of *Culex*—were drained. Old tires dotting the landscape, where mosquitoes bred in collected rainwater, became a thing of the past. Larvicide pellets were applied to other watery areas, such as New York City's one hundred thousand storm sewers, to kill the immature insects. Spraying also commenced to wipe out adult *C. pipiens*. Thousands of mosquitoes and birds were routinely collected and tested. As described in *Secret Agents* by Madeline Drexler, "In every borough (of NYC), white leghorn chickens deputized by the health department sat in secretly sited cages exposed to biting mosquitoes all spring and summer, bled each week by a veterinary technician to see if they had developed antibodies." New York is no third-world village, and emerging diseases are dealt with promptly and aggressively.

Yet West Nile continued to expand its mantle, cutting a swathe through twelve eastern states and Washington, D.C., sickening twenty-one and killing two in the spring and summer of 2000. By 2001 the virus struck animals and humans in the Deep South and Midwest. Experts predict that by 2006 the entire nation will play host to West Nile and that additional species of biting mosquitoes will transmit infection.

There is no prophylactic vaccine for humans and no specific treatment therapy for those infected. In more severe cases, intensive supportive therapy is indicated with intravenous feeding, ventilator support, and prevention of secondary infection. When frequenting mosquito-infested areas, the application of an insect repellent containing DEET should be considered, as well as the wearing of appropriate protective clothing (similar to the precautions recommended in Chapter 5, "New Kids on the Block," regarding Lyme disease). But you are in luck if you own a horse, since an equine vaccine does exist.

In retrospect, there are lessons to be learned from the handling of the West Nile outbreak by those involved in identifying the causative agent. For one thing, the CDC did not initially heed the warnings of veterinarians when they voiced concern over dying birds and suggested a possible link between their encephalitic deaths and the human encephalitis cases. The human illnesses were "presumptively" diagnosed as St. Louis encephalitis—the most widely reported mosquito-borne disease in the United States—when antibodies in patients' blood serum reacted with St. Louis virus in the lab. And St. Louis encephalitis does not kill birds, CDC researchers were quick to point out. But antibodies to related viruses will also react with the St. Louis strain, so the tests performed were not conclusive for St Louis. The debilitating disease could have been caused by another virus. CDC officials knew and chose to ignore this possibility. Weeks later they would realize their error and discover that the causative agent, far from being the garden-variety St. Louis bug, was one that had never before been seen—West Nile.

Legendary virus hunter J. C. Peters once offered this piece of wisdom to future epidemiologists, "When you hear hoofbeats in Central Park, think horses, not zebras." It is sound advice. First look for the obvious, since that will most likely be the cause of the event. But out of the corner of your eye, be watchful for the unusual, for the stripes on that horse. Be mindful that it is "on little cat's feet" that emerging germs and bioterror microbes may well steal into our lives and begin their deadly work. Once in a rare while those hoofbeats may be that of a zebra. And with bioterror and emerging infections on the rise, it might not be all that rare.

Why Viruses Emerge

Dengue, Ebola, Lassa, hantavirus, Marburg, West Nile—all are tropical or rain-forest viruses that have emerged recently as they made the cross-species jump from their natural hosts to humans. All have the potential to wreak havoc on humanity. One rain-forest virus in particular, HIV, has already begun realizing this potential. If scientists are to prevent global devastation and the human race is to escape a seemingly inevitable viral slaughter, it is imperative that we develop a very clear understanding of exactly how these killers come out of hiding.

As mentioned earlier, scientists do not generally believe that viruses suddenly start wiping out people because of spontaneous mutation or change in the virus. "Mutations," according to Robin Marantz Henig in her book *A Dancing Matrix: How Science Confronts Emerging Viruses*, "are almost never responsible for emerging viruses." Rather, it is a change in some human activity (like importing sick monkeys) or a natural disaster that unexpectedly allows the path of the virus to cross that of humans.

Global warming, for example, is creating new, hospitable habitats for virus-carrying mosquitoes and ticks. No longer confined to the tropics, they are exposing immunologically naive peoples to hitherto unknown deadly diseases. Floods and excessive rainfall present a similar problem, establishing new breeding grounds for insect vectors.

It is human activity, however, that most concerns virologists—activity such as destruction of the rain forests. For the last thirty years governments in South America and Africa have been engaging in a "slash and burn" campaign to clear rain forests for arable land—a well-meaning enterprise that unfortunately sends rain-forest animals scurrying in all directions, looking for new homes and new hosts. Crops that are subsequently planted, such as corn, only aggravate the problem, creating a dramatic increase in rodents. The result: epidemics of rodent-borne hemorrhagic fevers. Argentina and Bolivia experienced such outbreaks in the 1950s and early 1960s when grasslands were cleared and turned into farms.

Humans are learning the hard way that ecosystems are very fragile and delicately balanced. Tamper with them, and you open up a Pandora's box, the consequences of which can be dire and unpredictable. Consider the 1980 outbreak of Brazilian hemorrhagic fever—a story of viral emergence involving sand flies (also called biting midges), an occasionally fatal virus, and America's love of chocolate.

Chocolate first made its way to Europe in 1519, when the Spanish explorer Hernando Cortés brought it back with him from Mexico. Its popularity quickly spread, and when England began colonizing the New World chocolate became an early arrival to the shores of America. By 1980 the United States was consuming half the world's production of chocolate.

Such a demand did not go unnoticed by Brazil. Chocolate is made from the bean or seed of the cacao tree, a tropical plant that is indigenous to that country. Large pods that contain the beans are split open, and the beans and pulp are scooped out and allowed to ferment in the sun for about a week. The useless pods are discarded.

As more and more Brazilian farmers turned to cacao as a cash crop, empty pods began to pile up. Mountains of pods dotted the landscape, each pod collecting enough rainwater to serve as a breeding pool for the biting midges and the viruses they harbored. One virus to emerge, called *Oropouche*, caused a high-fever disease with a low mortality rate—Brazilian hemorrhagic fever.

On a much grander scale the building of dams has created huge bodies of standing water. Mosquitoes not normally found in a region invade the area and thrive in the dam-created floodlands. Such was the case with the Aswan High Dam in Egypt. Shortly after its construction (1971), Rift Valley fever, a deadly arboviral disease never before seen in Egypt, suddenly appeared and has caused periodic epidemics there ever since.

In many respects it seems as if life in the late twentieth and early twenty-first centuries is tailor-made for viral emergence. There is, for one thing, an unprecedented degree of human trafficking in third-world nations. Urbanization is causing an exodus from rural areas to large cities. Along with their baggage, people are bringing viruses from sparsely populated villages into crowded urban centers—and these centers are connected via air travel to every major world metropolis.

Political turmoil is also causing mass migration of humans. In 1972 Idi Amin ordered all Asians out of his country, effective immediately. Tens of thousands of Indians and other Asians fled not only Uganda but the entire continent of Africa. Many believe that the AIDS virus emerged from Uganda.

More recently, a brutal civil war between the Tutsis and Hutus in Rwanda has caused the largest short-term migration of refugees in history. More than a million Rwandans fled their homeland, pouring into Tanzania, Zaire, Uganda, and Burundi. Who knows what viruses were being transported throughout the continent? Or if any of those viruses happened to make it to an urban center? Or if any infected city dweller happened to make it onto an airplane headed for New York or London or . . . ? You get the picture. That is what's so terrifying. Any mysterious virus can hop a plane and be anywhere on the globe in a matter of hours. A person may sow the seeds of a pandemic before even realizing he or she is sick.

Which brings us to the creation of new and even deadlier germs—superbugs. As you will learn in Chapter 11, "Bioterrorism," scientists have intentionally manipulated the genetic material of germs to make them ever-more-efficient killers. But unbeknownst to medical practitioners, they may also have inadvertently created a situation in which novel and highly lethal viruses can develop naturally—inside immunosuppressed individuals.

People are usually given drugs to suppress their immune systems for one of two reasons: either as treatment for an autoimmune disease such as lupus or multiple sclerosis or as therapy following transplant surgery. Certain cancer treatments also compromise the immune system. The medications are essential if the procedures are to be successful. But they have also created a golden opportunity for viruses. Immune-suppressed people are easy targets for viral assault. Many often become infected with two or more viruses simultaneously. This is dangerous, for it allows the viruses, if they share the same cell and have similar nucleic acids, to swap genes, creating new, never-before-seen strains. If one virus happens to be extremely communicable and another extremely lethal, a mixing and matching of their genes could produce a hell of a hybrid.

Although this nightmare virus has not yet arisen, with all the immune systems out there that have been compromised by HIV, some virologists feel it is just a matter of time. Meanwhile, there is one common virus that routinely swaps genes with its cousins inside ducks and pigs. Usually not much comes out of these exchanges, but in 1917 a monster strain was born. Easily spread and very deadly, it swept across the globe, killing many in its path. In six months more than twenty million people perished; it is the closest humanity has come, thus far, to total annihilation. The disease? Influenza.

8

Common Viruses That Kill

There is no mortal whom sorrow and disease do not touch.

—EURIPIDES

Influenza

One of the worst plagues ever to afflict humankind occurred in 1918. It made half the world's population sick as it swept across the planet and killed millions of people—estimates run as high as forty million—in a matter of months. No pandemic before or since has wiped out so many people in so short a time. So desperate did the situation become that the commissioner of public health in Chicago told police to arrest anyone sneezing in public. San Francisco passed a law forcing people to wear surgical masks over their mouths and noses in public. Violators were arrested as "mask-slackers."

This dread killer was *influenza*, a disease originally blamed on the "influence" of heavenly bodies. Yes, influenza—the flu. Who would have thought this common malady could be such a merciless slayer? Since 1918 there have been two other major influenza pandemics—in 1957 and

1968—neither one as severe as the 1918 devastation. Virologists are scared to death that early into the new millennium another one will occur. They feel we are already overdue. Even in a good year the flu and flu-related pneumonia takes between twenty thousand and forty thousand lives in the United States, making it the sixth leading cause of disease death. The source of all this suffering and loss of life? An average-sized virus with several unique properties.

In the preceding chapter we looked at viruses that have the potential to emerge from animal reservoirs and devastate humanity. Well, in many respects the influenza virus is constantly emerging—or shall I say reemerging? It has the ability to do that—to change sufficiently so the body reacts to it as a new virus. The greater the change, the less recognition by the body and the greater the risk for a global disaster. Let's see how the influenza virus can accomplish this.

To begin with, the influenza virus is an RNA virus. As such it has an uncommonly high mutation rate—up to one million times that of DNA. Only HIV, another RNA virus, mutates faster. When mutations occur, new viral particles get genes that are different from the parent particle. Different genes mean different coat proteins, and this is where the problem lies. If we were to be infected each year with the same strain of flu (same outer protein coat), the memory cells of our immune system would have no difficulty recognizing the invaders. A rapid, overwhelming antibody response would thwart the infection before it ever began. But even a slight variation of the outer viral coat could slow down recognition and response by the body. The enemy, approaching in disguise, could infiltrate our defenses and cause disease.

This is what typically happens from year to year. Flu bugs change just enough, through mutation, to slow down our immune response and cause another bout of influenza. Such minor changes in the virus, which cause yearly flu "epidemics," are called *antigenic drift*. (*Antigen* refers to the outer protein coat.)

The major pandemics that come along periodically and kill millions of people are not caused by the same errors of gene replication. Other forces dramatically alter the relatively benign virus and transform it into a monster—forces that involve pigs and ducks as well as genetic material that could pass for pasta salad.

If you were to observe the genetic material of a flu virus under a powerful electron microscope, it would look very much like pasta salad, with twists of macaroni entwined with one another. There would be eight twists or segments to be exact, each twist containing a portion of the genetic material. Two of these segments are of particular concern to virologists, for each contains a gene that makes a viral coat protein. It is these two coat proteins that act as antigens to which our immune system reacts, producing antibodies. Change either or both of these proteins, and you confound the system.

For simplicity's sake, let us call the two proteins, hemagglutinin and neuraminidase, by their first letters, H and N. Since 1933, when the first human flu virus was isolated, fourteen different subtypes of H antigen and nine subtypes of N antigen have been identified. Each subtype of H or N is radically different from any other subtype. Antibodies against one subtype will not react with another.

Such major changes in the H or N protein of a virus do not come about through one or even several simple mutations. Errors of replication during infection will not transform one subtype into another. For this to occur there must actually be a swapping of RNA segments between different viral strains. Enter the ducks and pigs.

Influenza viruses that infect humans also feel very much at home in pigs and ducks and other water birds. Many birds, in fact, are simultaneously infected with several different strains of flu. Usually the virus thrives in the digestive tract and causes no ill effects. It is believed that all the genes of all the different strains of flu viruses are being maintained in the bellies of ducks and other aquatic fowl.

Now imagine, if you will, two different strains of flu virus growing inside the cell of a duck. When the RNA segments replicate and sort into different viral particles, there can be a mixing and matching of the segments. A virus might get six segments from one strain and two segments from the other. If the genetic reshuffling happens to involve the segment containing the H or N gene, a new strain with radically different surface antigens can be produced. Such a sudden and severe change is called *antigenic shift*. If the recombinant strain is capable of infecting and causing illness in humans, a new pandemic looms on the horizon.

It has been shown experimentally that reassortment of viral genes into novel combinations does indeed occur in ducks. But virologists believe it is the pig that is nature's true mixing vessel for flu viruses. Pigs are multiply infected quite readily with all sorts of flu viruses from both ducks and humans. It would be no trouble at all for a human flu bug, replicating inside a pig cell, to be dealt an H or N gene from a duck strain. The 1918 flu—commonly known as the Spanish flu—was in fact caused by a variety of virus that came to be called the *swine flu*. More about the swine flu later.

The flu virus is very much like my wife—every year she gets a new coat. Now that scientists have deduced the mechanism by which that coat is made, it should not be very difficult to correct the problem. Simply keep ducks and pigs and humans away from one another as much as possible. If different strains are not given the opportunity to coinfect a host, no superflu bugs can be created. Easier said than done, especially in China, Taiwan, and other Asian countries, where farming practices bring these animals into close contact with one another. In an agricultural technique known as *polyculture*, hens are kept in cages hung above pigs, which feed on the hen droppings. Fresh pig feces are, in turn, used to fertilize fish ponds, where ducks swim, drink, and eliminate their own wastes. The practice is a very economical way of increasing yields of high-protein foods such as fish. These yields, however, come at a price. Each year some new flu strain emerges from these Asian farms—Hong Kong flu or Shanghai flu or Singapore flu or Bangkok flu—and makes its way around the globe. Luckily there has been no epidemic strain since 1968, but creation of such a bug is an accident waiting to happen. Meanwhile scientists around the world are on a constant vigil, swabbing and culturing throats of sick humans and animals, awaiting Armageddon. In 1976 they feared the dreaded superflu had arrived when a healthy nineteen-year-old army recruit at Fort Dix, New Jersey, died of influenza.

The Swine Flu Scare of 1976

The story begins on February 4, 1976. Private David Lewis, stationed at the Fort Dix army base in New Jersey, was suffering from a bout of flu. Nonetheless, he foolishly went on a five-mile march in the dead of winter. Following the march, suffering from high fever and respiratory distress, he collapsed and died. Young, healthy men do not usually succumb to influenza, so throat washings from David as well as eighteen other patients were sent to the CDC for analysis. Tests were run on the swabs to see what known flu antibodies they reacted with. This would identify the subtype of flu strain present in the sputum—what H and N antigens studded the virus's surface. Most of the results were what doctors expected, a form of H3N2 flu virus—the type that caused the pandemic of 1968. Since then antigenic drift variations of the H3N2 virus had been circulating the planet, causing typically mild outbreaks every year or so. Five samples, however, alarmed the experts. They reacted with antibodies to an H1N1 virus—the swine flu bug responsible for the 1918 horror. The 1918 virus had been given the moniker swine flu way back in the 1930s, when it was shown to react with antibodies made against a pig flu virus. Not since 1918, however, had H1N1 been seen in human populations. Now, sixty years later, it was reappearing, and humanity, immunologically naive and susceptible after nearly sixty years of nonexposure, would be ill prepared.

In every way measurable the Fort Dix H1N1 strain was indistinguishable from the 1918 killer strain. What a sobering discovery. Thoughts immediately focused on a vaccine to protect the population against impending doom. Vaccines against specific subtypes of influenza had been made in the past, and the technology was there. Large quantities of the virus had to be grown in huge vats and then attenuated. But it was expensive and time-consuming to produce enough vaccine for an entire nation. Additionally, there was the risk of people reacting negatively to the vaccine itself. Decisions had to be made and made quickly. On March 24, less than two months after the Fort Dix casualty, President Gerald Ford met with a blue-ribbon panel of the world's top virologists. Doctors Jonas Salk and Albert Sabin of polio vaccine fame were both there. The president wanted to know whether the dangers were imminent enough to warrant a nationwide vaccination program. None in the room counseled against vaccination. Later that evening Ford went on television to recommend that Congress appropriate funds for a vaccination program for all Americans. By mid-April a bill was passed by Congress and signed by the president. Some 196 million doses of vaccine were to be manufactured at a cost of $135 million by November 1.

In the meantime, many experts were having second thoughts. Since the death of Private Lewis the potential slate-wiper seemed to be causing few problems. It appeared as if the virus, although passable from pigs to humans, was not easily spread from person to person. Perhaps there was overreaction on the part of the scientific and medical community. Then, in

July of that year, a mysterious flulike disease struck 221 people who had attended an American Legion convention in Philadelphia. It turned out to be Legionnaires' disease (discussed in Chapter 5, "New Kids on the Block") and was totally unrelated to swine flu. Nonetheless it greatly escalated fears about a potential massive swine flu outbreak. Any hesitation on the part of politicians evaporated, and the vaccination program continued full steam ahead. On October 1, 1976, at the Indiana State Fair, the first swine flu shots were given.

Ten days later three people who had received the swine flu vaccine suddenly died. By October 14, the number had climbed to more than a dozen. People were coming down with a rare neurological disorder called Guillain-Barré syndrome, apparently triggered by the swine flu vaccination. As casualties continued to mount, the CDC called a halt to the swine flu campaign. It seemed to be doing more harm than good, especially in light of the fact that no one was contracting H1N1 influenza. The dreaded pandemic never materialized because the virus never really made it out of the pig population.

In retrospect the 1976 swine flu vaccination initiative was a monumental blunder. The virus, although H1N1, was different in subtle ways from the ultravirulent strain that had devastated humanity six decades earlier. Most significantly, it was not nearly as transmissible. But, smitten with swine flu hysteria, the experts launched America on an expensive, unnecessary, and, on rare occasions, dangerous campaign of mass inoculation. Some unfairly blamed Gerald Ford for the fiasco, a perception that may have cost him the presidency as he lost a reelection bid to Jimmy Carter in November of that year.

Meanwhile, pigs and ducks continue to play musical genes with the influenza virus. One day this random mixing and matching will inadvertently produce the easily transmissible, highly virulent superbug that made scientists so paranoid two-and-a-half decades ago. Let's hope we will be up to the challenge when that day arrives.

The ABCs of Hepatitis

In 1895, 1,300 workers at a shipyard in Germany were vaccinated against smallpox. The vaccine was administered by placing a drop, prepared from human blood serum, onto the skin and then scratching the skin with a needle. Very likely the same needle was used many times without proper sterilization. A few months later 191 of the workers developed a sickly yellow coloration of the skin—jaundice. Jaundice occurs when the liver does not destroy old red blood cells properly, producing a greenish-yellow pigment called *bilirubin*.

In 1942, with America deeply entrenched in World War II, the Rockefeller Institute mass-produced several million doses of a new yellow fever vaccine. The vaccine, also prepared using human blood serum, was intended to immunize army recruits stationed in the Philippines. Shortly after vaccination, however, thirty thousand soldiers complained of fever, headache, chills, vomiting, loss of appetite, and extreme fatigue, soon followed by jaundice. Eighty-four of the recruits died.

In both tragedies a vaccine administered to prevent one viral disease inadvertently caused another: hepatitis B.

Hepatitis comes in several different forms, the most important being hepatitis A, hepatitis B, and hepatitis C. All infect and damage the liver; *hepatitis*, in fact, means "liver inflammation." They are, however, caused by very disparate viruses.

Hepatitis A

Hepatitis A is spread orally when contaminated food or water is ingested. Inadequate sewage disposal and unclean living conditions enable the hepatitis A virus to thrive. It is a disease of feces and filth. Mussels and clams growing in polluted waters often harbor the virus. Although there are no longer broad epidemics of hepatitis A in the United States, in 1971 it did strike fifty thousand Americans. Today outbreaks occur mainly in day-care centers.

Thankfully, it is the mildest form of hepatitis, and people usually recover from the disease's nausea, vomiting, black urine, and jaundice in a month or two. A vaccine consisting of inactivated virus is also available and recommended before travel in some parts of the world. There are no chronic cases of hepatitis A and no lifetime carriers. It is an acute infection, and recovery means complete elimination of the virus.

Hepatitis B

Regrettably this is not the case with hepatitis B. It is caused by a very different virus (HBV) with a very different mode of infection. To begin with, transmission occurs through sexual contact and contact with contaminated blood and body fluids. In this respect it is much like HIV, although HBV is one hundred times more infectious than the AIDS virus. Like HIV, it causes a serious, often deadly disease.

Hepatitis B infects 5 percent of the world's population with a lifelong, chronic infection, in which the virus is tolerated by the immune system. That's a whopping 300 million people, 1.25 million of whom are Americans. In areas of Southeast Asia and tropical Africa and among gay men and intravenous drug users the percentages are much higher. Long-term infection and destruction of liver cells leads in many cases to cirrhosis. It is estimated that globally, one million people die annually from hepatitis B. Chronic HBV infection also causes five million cases of liver cancer each year. As a proven cancer-causing agent, hepatitis B ranks second only to cigarettes in number of fatalities.

Given these gruesome statistics, it is not surprising that in the year 2000 the WHO considered hepatitis B one of the world's deadliest scourges. Only tuberculosis, AIDS, and malaria as distinct infectious diseases had a higher kill rate (see Table 3). The tragedy of it all is that an effective vaccine against hepatitis B has existed since 1981. All that remains is to get the vaccine (a series of three inoculations over a six-month period) to the half billion people who need it.

Development of the hepatitis B vaccine did not come easily. It was the culmination of a twenty-five-year wrestling match with the elusive virus. And the first to enter the ring against the microbe was Dr. Saul Krugman.

Table 3 *The World's Deadliest Scourges—Year 2000*

Infectious Disease	Cause	Annual Deaths
acute respiratory infections (mostly pneumonia)	bacterial or viral	more than 4 million
diarrheal diseases of varied etiology	bacterial, viral, or protozoan	more than 3 million
tuberculosis	bacterial	3 million (about half coinfected with HIV)
AIDS	viral	3 million (up from .7 million in 1993)
malaria	protozoan	1–2 million (probably nearer the higher figure)
hepatitis B	viral	1 million
measles	viral	.8 million

The story begins in 1955. Dr. Krugman, professor of pediatrics at New York University Medical School, received a call from the Willowbrook State School for the Retarded. Located on 375 acres in Staten Island, Willowbrook's twenty-four buildings housed four thousand of New York State's most severely retarded children. Conditions in the facility were deplorable. There was overcrowding and filth everywhere. Children were literally eating each other's feces. Not surprisingly, hepatitis was running rampant, and virtually every child was infected. What, if anything, could be done to ameliorate the situation?

Dr. Krugman embarked on an eleven-year odyssey of experimentation that was as controversial as it was enlightening. With parental consent, he both fed and injected hepatitis-contaminated blood serums into newly admitted patients. Attempting to learn more about the disease, he discovered that two viruses were at play in Willowbrook, each causing a distinct disease. One was spread orally and the other through blood contact. Immunity to one did not confer immunity to the other. In short, the good doctor had identified hepatitis A and hepatitis B. The viral foe had suddenly become a tag team.

Not to worry. Dr. Krugman had a tag team partner of his own, Dr. Baruch Blumberg. Working at the National Institutes of Health (NIH), Blumberg was involved in research having absolutely nothing to do with hepatitis. He was collecting and analyzing blood from different racial groups throughout the world to isolate new proteins. Hopefully these proteins would be indicative of genetic differences that made one population more or less susceptible to a disease than another.

What Dr. Blumberg found one glorious day in 1963 was a completely novel and unexpected protein in the blood of a hemophiliac. Hemophiliacs lack a certain clotting factor in their blood called *Factor VIII*. As a result, their blood clots very slowly. Today microbes can mass-produce this factor through the miracle of genetic engineering. Such technology, however, did not exist in the sixties—or the seventies for that matter. To get enough Factor VIII to inject into a "bleeder," the blood of thousands of people had to be pooled. It is estimated that a typical hemophiliac was annually exposed to the blood of more than two million donors. Blumberg therefore assumed, and correctly, that this never-before-seen protein was an antibody the hemophiliac was making in response to some antigen he had received in a transfusion.

The newfound antibody, when tested against other blood serums, reacted only with that of an Australian aborigine. What possible antigen could an Australian possess that a New York hemophiliac would have made antibodies against?

That was what Blumberg and his associates wanted to know. They started testing blood in earnest, looking everywhere for the Australian antigen (dubbed *Au*). Although it is rare in the general American population, individuals with leukemia and Down's syndrome commonly showed the presence of Au. The scientists were at a loss to explain their findings.

Then, early in 1966, something strange happened. A Down's patient who had tested negative for Au was found to be positive on a subsequent blood test. Furthermore, tests of liver function revealed that he had come down with hepatitis. At last the pieces of the jigsaw puzzle were beginning to fall into place. Au must be an antigen associated with hepatitis, possibly the virus itself. It turned up so often in people with Down's syndrome and in patients with hemophilia and leukemia because of the large number of transfusions they received—transfusions that infected them with hepatitis!

Further confirmation came later in 1966, when one of Blumberg's lab technicians contracted hepatitis. A blood test for the Au antigen was quickly performed. Sure enough, her blood, which had previously tested negative, suddenly came back positive.

Now Blumberg contacted Krugman and asked for samples of his hepatitis A– and hepatitis B–infected blood. Would they show presence of the Au antigen? One, the hepatitis B blood, did. Au, it turned out, was an antigen on the surface of hepatitis B viral particles.

At last the hepatitis B virus had been pinned to the mat. This meant that almost immediately a screening test for donated blood could be developed and put to use. By 1973 such screening became mandatory in American blood banks.

Unfortunately, the production and distribution of a successful vaccine took a while longer. The main stumbling block was the virus's exceeding reluctance to grow in the laboratory. In another respect, however, researchers were very lucky in their dealings with hepatitis B. Unlike any other virus, when it grew in human cells it produced trillions of smaller, noninfectious particles. They were noninfectious because they contained no nucleic acid, although their surfaces were crawling with a viral surface antigen. It was like a godsend—particles that could elicit a strong immune response but were not infectious. The perfect vaccine.

Scientists succeeded in collecting and purifying these antigen particles from the blood of patients with chronic hepatitis B. They became the stuff of the first hepatitis B vaccine—and arguably the first cancer vaccine. Extreme efforts were undertaken to kill any other possible contaminants that might be present in the blood serum. We are very fortunate that such extraordinary precautions were taken, since HIV, which had not been discovered yet, was most assuredly circulating in the blood pool by that time (mid- to late 1970s).

Today the surface antigen is produced more cheaply and safely through genetic engineering. The gene for the surface antigen is snipped out of the virus and placed in yeast cells. Here it spews large quantities of antigen that can be harvested from the culture medium. Another triumph for science. As already mentioned, all that remains is delivery of the vaccine to the half billion people who need it. In the United States alone, only 1 percent of the millions of people at risk have received the vaccine. The National Foundation for Infectious Diseases, in an attempt to reverse these statistics, has been running public service announcements emphasizing the importance of hepatitis B prevention. In May 2001 the Food and Drug Administration approved a vaccine called Twinrix against hepatitis A and B for people over age eighteen.

As a footnote, there is some concern about giving the vaccine uniformly to all children and young adults, since the inoculations have been associated, in rare instances, with symptoms of multiple sclerosis and arthritis. Some feel that only youngsters in jeopardy of contracting hepatitis B should be given the vaccine.

Hepatitis C

By the late 1970s scientists were finding that a sizable number of their hepatitis patients were testing negative for both the A and B viruses. They began wringing their hands, afraid that a new virus was at work. Their fears were well founded. A new agent was responsible for the mysterious liver ailments. Although first labeled *hepatitis non-A, non-B*, once the causative agent was isolated in 1989, it was renamed *hepatitis C (HCV)*.

Like hepatitis B, hepatitis C is transmitted through body fluids. And like hepatitis B, it is a bad one, killing and disabling millions each year. Although it is not yet as common globally as hepatitis B, a much higher percentage of hepatitis C sufferers become chronically infected, leading to cirrhosis and liver cancer. It is the most common blood-borne infection in the United States, with nearly four million Americans infected. Ten thousand died in 2001, which was twice the number of hepatitis B fatalities. Hepatitis C is the leading cause of liver transplants in the United States. Country singer Naomi Judd and model/actress Pamela Anderson are living with HCV. Thankfully there is a screening test for donated blood, but a prophylactic vaccine does not exist, so the figures of those infected will likely increase. Hepatitis C virus simply replicates too fast—one hundred trillion new particles produced daily—creating such viral diversity that vaccines become useless. A typical patient may have fifteen to twenty variants of a single subtype of HCV, and there are 150 different subtypes.

The antiviral drugs interferon, injected three times a week for six to twelve months and given in conjunction with ribavirin, is most commonly used to fight the hepatitis C virus. It is effective if started within two to three months of infection. Early diagnosis and treatment is critical. Meanwhile, new antivirals are being investigated. In one novel approach call *pegylation*, molecules of polyethylene glycol (PEG) are bonded to interferon. The "pegylated" interferons are harder for the body to flush out, allowing the medication to remain in a patient's system for up to seven days instead of the usual forty-eight hours. This reduces the number of weekly injections from three to one, diminishing the likelihood of side effects such as flulike symptoms, hair loss, depression, and anemia. As a result, patients can remain in drug therapy longer. And still the quest for a vaccine continues.

Alphabet Soup

For the purists, let me just add that the string of hepatitis infections does not end with hepatitis C. There is a D, for delta virus, which is found only in coinfections with hepatitis B. When delta factor is present, hepatitis B symptoms become much more acute and severe. Luckily the hepatitis B vaccine will also wipe out delta infection.

Hepatitis E virus (HEV) causes a disease similar to hepatitis A and is acute rather than chronic. It is spread through fecal contamination of hands, food, water, or raw shellfish. Although hepatitis E is unusual in the United States, the virus has produced large outbreaks in Asia and South America. In the early and mid-1990s two new viruses were isolated and identified that brought about infection with liver involvement. This ran the string of hepatitis viruses to G.

The apparent unending discovery of new hepatitis viruses should not be considered extraordinary. It is estimated that we have not yet identified 90 percent of the animals that roam this planet, so why should the finding of an unknown virus come as such a shock? Scientists believe we know virtually nothing about 95 percent of the roughly five thousand species of viruses that exist. Of the approximately one million species of bacteria, we have characterized about two thousand. There will, undoubtedly, be many more surprises.

Poliomyelitis (Infantile Paralysis)

Polio first became epidemic in the United States in 1916 and for almost four decades struck fear in the hearts of America's mothers and fathers. During that time it annually crippled and killed up to forty thousand children.

Few diseases have caused the public concern that infantile paralysis did in the first half of this century. Flu, an illness that killed more people in one year (1918) than polio did in twenty-five, did not instill such dread. Every summer parents shuddered at the thought of their children swimming, picnicking, going to the movies, playing with friends. For it was in those months that the frightful disease struck with a vengeance.

Polio, like hepatitis A, is spread when contaminated substances are swallowed—water from a swimming pool, for example. The virus invades cells of the intestine and multiplies rapidly. The vast majority of polio infections remain in the gut and cause no serious problems, often going totally unnoticed. But now and again the virus makes its way out of the digestive tract and to the nervous system, where it begins killing off neurons. When this happens, paralysis is a frequent outcome.

That poliovirus initially infects cells of the gut and not nerve cells wasn't realized until 1948, when Dr. John Enders grew poliovirus in a tissue culture of mouse intestine. It won him the 1954 Nobel Prize in Physiology or Medicine. It also provided Dr. Jonas Salk with the knowledge he needed to grow poliovirus in his laboratory.

Dr. Salk, along with Dr. Albert Sabin and a number of other researchers, was hoping to develop a polio vaccine. Armed now with the appropriate tissue cultures, he began growing the virus. Actually there were three separate strains of poliovirus that needed culturing. Afterward Salk killed the viruses with formalin, a chemical commonly used to preserve dead animals. Once inactivated, the mixture of dead viruses was incorporated into a vaccine— a vaccine that, in April 1955, was licensed and distributed to millions of Americans.

The Salk vaccine proved remarkably effective. From nearly thirty thousand new cases a year figures dropped to under one thousand. Dr. Salk became an instant celebrity. He was showered with honors and gifts. President Dwight Eisenhower presented him with a special citation at the White House. Hollywood even wanted to film his life story, with Marlon Brando possibly playing the lead.

But then, in the late 1950s, polio seemed to reemerge, with more than eight thousand new cases in 1959. The reason was simple. Many of the country's poorest children, those who needed it most, were not being vaccinated.

Sabin, always the opportunist, seized the moment to hawk his own vaccine, a live but attenuated mixture of poliovirus strains. He claimed that his version of the polio vaccine would be more effective in wiping out this crippling plague. Most of the scientific community agreed with him.

Unlike the Salk vaccine, which was injected, Sabin's was dripped onto a sugar cube and then eaten—or mixed into an orange-flavored drink. The virus, weakened through continued growth in monkey-kidney tissue, actually infected cells of the human intestine. Here the immune system fought the virus, conferring lifelong immunity (Salk's vaccine was not lifelong, and repeated booster shots were required). Because of its attenuation, Sabin's vaccine was unable to infect nerve cells. It therefore provided immunity with no risk of paralysis or death. And since it was a living virus, it could be transmitted through natural channels to friends and family members. In this way the Sabin vaccine offered more widespread immunity to the population as a whole. As a final selling point, the Sabin vaccine was cheaper and easier to manufacture.

Enough said. All things considered, the United States opted for the Sabin oral polio vaccine (OPV), and by the early 1960s it was being used almost exclusively throughout most of the globe. Over the years it has virtually wiped out polio in the Western world. But OPV has one serious drawback. On very rare occasions it reverts or mutates back to a virulent form. Remember, we are dealing with live viruses. This results in about eight to ten children each year developing polio from the oral, live-virus vaccine. These vaccine-associated polios led the CDC in the year 2000 to change vaccination policy, eliminating use of oral polio vaccine in favor of the killed-virus injections.

So successful has mass immunization been that in September 1994 the Pan American Health Organization announced the eradication of polio in the Western Hemisphere. Yet something was afoot. Polio survivors, many who had conquered the disease thirty-odd years earlier, were suddenly experiencing fatigue, pain, and muscle weakness. The numbers were too great to be ignored. Roughly one-third of the 1.5 million survivors were coming down with what came to be called *postpolio syndrome* (*PPS*).

At first it was believed that the initial infection robbed the body of too many motor neurons. When additional nerve cells were lost in old age, it was the proverbial straw that broke the camel's back. A similar theory held that remaining nerves and/or muscles that had been "overworked" for years were failing prematurely. Then researchers reported evidence of poliovirus fragments in the spinal fluid of PPS sufferers. Could the virus have survived in nerve cells all those years, only now destroying the individual nerve terminals of motor neurons? As this book goes to print, scientists cannot agree on the significance of the findings and continue to investigate this strange turn of events.

Regrettably, the great success the polio vaccine has enjoyed in North America and Europe is not reflected through the rest of the world. Polio virus still lurks in south Asia and sub-Saharan Africa where it is a dangerous crippler, bringing pain and paralysis to thirty-five hundred children in twenty countries and infecting hundreds of thousands more in the year 2000. But efforts are being made by WHO, UNICEF, and the CDC to effect global eradication by 2005. It will not be easy. Countries such as Sudan, Somalia, Afghanistan, Angola, and the Democratic Republic of Congo are plagued with internal conflict, making implementation of vaccination surveillance activities particularly challenging. It will take a massive initiative on the scale employed to eliminate smallpox from the planet. Such an effort could also wipe out measles, a disease that currently kills many more people worldwide than polio. Measles, however, like influenza, is the Rodney Dangerfield of disease: it gets no respect.

Measles

Measles is very possibly the most contagious virus on Earth, although cold and flu sufferers might argue the point. According to Ann Giudici Fettner, author of *The Science of Viruses*, "A child can catch measles by breathing the air in a doctor's waiting room two hours after an infected child has left." So incredibly transmissible is the virus that if one infected person entered a town or village of several thousand immunologically naive people, within six weeks virtually 100 percent of the susceptible population would have caught it. This is precisely what happened to the Eskimos of Greenland when measles struck there in 1951. Dr. Georges Peter, chair of the American Academy of Pediatrics, calls measles "the most contagious of all vaccine-preventable diseases."

As mentioned in the Introduction, measles was one of the diseases that Europeans brought with them to the New World—one of the diseases that wiped out the Native Americans. The Eskimos of Greenland were devastated by the disease. Even today measles kills on a grand scale. Worldwide it strikes about thirty million children each year and kills nearly one million of them, making it, as a distinct infectious illness, one of the most prevalent causes of juvenile death. Along with hepatitis B, measles is the most lethal of all vaccine-preventable diseases. Hardest hit, by far, are the developing countries, where it is among the deadliest of scourges, right up there with malaria, tuberculosis, and AIDS.

The Western world has fared much better. Even before the development of a vaccine, it was never the killer it was—and still is—in third-world countries. It was a nuisance illness for the half million Americans who contracted the disease annually—a rite of passage through childhood. Only on rare occasions did it affect the brain and cause coma and death. Even so, this uncommon complication led to several hundred to a thousand deaths a year in America alone. In 1963 a vaccine was developed that essentially eliminated this threat to developed nations.

The sad part is that measles could be completely eliminated from the planet. The vaccines for both measles and polio are extremely effective, and, most important, neither disease occurs in animals other than humans. We are the only natural reservoir. This is critical for eradication of a disease. It is the reason yellow fever, influenza, and rabies, other deadly viral diseases, cannot be wiped out while smallpox could. There will always be wild animals that harbor these viruses—animals eager to share their microbes with us.

But as with smallpox, the effort must be worldwide. We cannot eliminate measles from the West and have it running rampant in Africa and Asia. We are, after all, a global community. Although measles is a rarity in America today, due to improved vaccines and a rigorous inoculation campaign, it can come roaring back at any time. It did in fact come roaring back in 1989 and 1990, when about fifty thousand cases turned up, resulting in about a hundred deaths. The resurgence, from an all-time low in 1983, was due to a slackening of the vaccine vigil, especially in poor urban areas.

A final note on the dangers of allowing the measles virus or any other microbe to hang around: in time germs mutate—they change into other strains. Sometimes these strains are more virulent, more lethal. Often the antibodies we possess from vaccination with the garden-variety virus will not react with the new strain. In other words, we are susceptible to the new bug. We see this happening with flu viruses every year. Thankfully measles and most other viruses are not as mutable, and the same vaccine is effective year after year. But even with stable viruses we should not press our luck. In 1995 a new virus closely related to measles did appear in Australia, where it killed a rancher and about a dozen horses by causing the lungs to fill with blood.

Unfortunately, measles does most of its damage in countries that are too poor to initiate eradication programs, and richer countries have no desire to allocate huge sums of money to fight third-world diseases. This is a problem not only with measles but with many other diseases as well. Chief among the illnesses that receive little attention from developed nations, even though they kill and maim untold millions, are those caused by parasites.

9

Parasites That Kill

Disease is not of the body, but of the place.

—SENECA

EPIDEMIOLOGISTS ARE BIOLOGICAL sleuths called in when epidemics strike to try to ascertain how and why they occurred. Robin Marantz Henig makes the interesting observation in her book *A Dancing Matrix* that, were a seasoned African epidemiologist to be asked, "What constitutes an epidemic worth looking into?" he would most likely answer, "The death of one white person."

Life is cheaper in third-world countries than in developed nations. Preventable diseases that incapacitate and kill hundreds of millions of people throughout Africa, Asia, and Central and South America are allowed to run amok. The World Health Organization (WHO) estimated that in 1998 two billion children suffered acute respiratory infections and more than four million died—the vast majority in emerging countries. Eighty percent of these deaths were due to bacterial lung infections, largely preventable or curable, such as pneumonia. Much of the world's population still suffers and dies from diseases contracted through unclean water. These include bacterial and viral diarrheas as well as diseases caused by parasites.

Every year 1.7 billion people suffer from infections acquired through water contaminated by parasites or their animal hosts.

Strictly speaking, a parasite is an organism that lives on or in another organism upon which it feeds. By definition, then, bacteria and viruses are parasites, and the diseases they cause are parasitic diseases. Traditionally, however, biologists have used the term *parasite* in a more limited sense, to refer to larger, more complex living things, such as protozoa and worms. And tradition is hard to break. Even today the designation *parasite* is usually meant to exclude viruses and bacteria.

Protozoa

Once believed to be tiny animals because they are motile and not green, protozoa now belong to their own distinct kingdom. They are the simplest of the parasites. Although bacteria and protozoa are both one-celled organisms, the cell of a protozoan is larger and vastly more complex. Anyone who has taken biology in high school has seen protozoa under a microscope. They include the often-studied amoeba and paramecium. Protozoa are ubiquitous, being found in virtually any watery environment—ponds, rivers, lakes, fish tanks.

Most protozoa are free-living—they have no hosts—and cause people and other animals no harm. Unfortunately several are parasitic, and a few present very serious health problems to infected individuals. Way back in 1875 a protozoan was first shown to be a pathogen. It was *Entamoeba histolytica*, the dysentery amoeba familiar to anyone foolish enough to drink unbottled water in countries lacking proper sewage disposal. Two hundred years before that, the great microscopist Antonie van Leeuwenhoek noticed a protozoan flitting about in his feces. It was a "wee animalcule" of the *Giardia* genus. Since Leeuwenhoek's discovery, *Giardia lamblia* and another protozoan, *Cryptosporidium*, have been implicated in many outbreaks of painful intestinal infections and severe diarrhea worldwide. They are found routinely in drinking water that has been polluted by human or animal feces. In April 1993, four hundred thousand Milwaukee residents came down with cryptosporidiosis; forty-four hundred were hospitalized. It seems that the protozoan is resistant to standard chlorination procedures used for drinking water and can, in fact, survive in full-strength Clorox. Chalk one up for the microbes.

Intestinal parasites aside, it is the bite of tropical insects that spreads the worst protozoan diseases—those that continue to plague third-world countries.

Sleeping Sickness (African Trypanosomiasis)

Sleeping sickness is one such deadly disease, caused by a small fishlike protozoan called a *trypanosome*, which swims in the blood by lashing a whiplike tail or *flagellum*. The illness is transmitted through the bite of a tsetse fly and eventually leads to loss of consciousness and death when the organisms invade the spinal cord and brain. Sleeping sickness is also a disease of livestock such as cattle, and in many areas where the disease is endemic it can literally wipe out the homegrown meat supply. Some experts feel that global warming can greatly expand the habitats of tsetse flies, prevalent throughout Africa, and hence the distribution of the disease they carry. In general global warming is threatening to expand the territories of many insect vectors.

Leishmaniasis

In the year 2000 there were twelve million cases of leishmaniasis worldwide. It is a debilitating and often fatal affliction caused by the leishmania protozoan—an organism "no weightier than an eyelash," to quote noted parasitologist Robert Desowitz. And the insect that brings this deadly scourge to humanity, a tiny blood-sucking sand fly, is not much weightier than an eyelash. But the two team up to produce epidemics that kill hundreds of thousands of people in India, China, northern Africa, and Brazil.

The most deadly form of the disease is visceral leishmaniasis, also called *kala-azar*. It has wiped out two-thirds of some hard-hit villages. The symptoms of kala-azar are unremitting fever, skin that turns dark gray, severe anemia, and a spleen and liver that are grossly enlarged, distending the abdomen. If left untreated the disease has a mortality rate approaching 100 percent. Leishmania protozoa actually live inside white blood cells that should swallow up and kill the protozoa. They do swallow them up but are unable to finish the job. The leishmania protozoa, in fact, thrive inside white blood cells. Over time they destroy these cells and, much like HIV, wreak havoc on the immune system. A depressed immune system allows other deadly bacterial infections such as pneumonia or dysentery to overcome the body's defenses. Speaking of HIV, this deadly virus has been found increasingly coinfecting people along with the leishmania protozoan. Although most people bitten by leishmania-carrying sand flies do not develop disease, coinfection with HIV quickly evolves into severe leishmaniasis.

The standard treatment for leishmaniasis is an intravenous therapy using highly poisonous antimony compounds. If the disease doesn't kill the patient, the cure will. Recently another, safer drug—miltefosine—administered orally has proven effective in animal tests. A possible vaccine also looms on the horizon. Then again, the mere possession of a successful vaccine means very little as diseases such as measles dramatically demonstrate.

It has even been suggested that leishmaniasis did in the dinosaurs. Although not overly compelling, the evidence cannot be dismissed summarily. Remember *Jurassic Park*, a clever bit of science fiction in which dinosaurs were cloned using preserved insects that had sucked the blood of dinosaurs some seventy or eighty million years earlier? Dinosaurs, of course, cannot be cloned, but the fossil record reveals that they were indeed parasitized by insects, several species of which were sand flies. And DNA comparison of different leishmania species (some of which infect lizards) indicates that they also have been evolving for about eighty million years. It is therefore not unreasonable to speculate that prehistoric sand flies harbored leishmania protozoa that they injected into dinosaurs. If this is true, and it contributed to dinosaur extinction, then we owe quite a lot to the sand fly and leishmania protozoan, for it was extinction of the dinosaurs that allowed primitive mammals and eventually humans to evolve.

Malaria

The word *malaria* means "bad air," air that, according to the ancient Greeks, made people deathly ill with intermittent fever. But no one at the time could identify the precise cause of illness. Hippocrates believed miasmas—deadly mists—were at play, somehow upsetting the balance of the body's four humors: blood, phlegm, black bile, and yellow bile. Sound silly? Well, the ancient Chinese attributed paroxysmal fever—malaria—to an imbalance or disharmony between the yin and yang, two opposing life forces in the body. And the great taxonomist Carolus Linnaeus, to whom we owe the genus-species method of scientifically naming organisms, hypothesized that tiny suspended particles of clay in drinking water clogged blood vessels, thereby bringing on the disease. Not until 1898 would the true cause of malaria be identified—the bite of a mosquito infected with a deadly protozoan.

That protozoan is *Plasmodium falciparum*, and it might well kill more humans than any other pathogen . . . save perhaps the bacillus of tuberculosis or the AIDS virus. Malaria is endemic throughout most of the world, but because so many deaths occur in third-world countries, annual fatality figures are rough estimates at best. Even so, the loss of life is staggering, somewhere between one and two million people, probably closer to the latter. Perhaps three hundred million people are diagnosed each year with clinical malaria. In severely malarious areas people are bitten several hundred times a year by *Plasmodium*-infected mosquitoes. Contracting the disease is almost inevitable. Robert Desowitz, in his book *The Malaria Capers*, offers us a vivid description of a young pregnant woman in the throes of a malarial "rigor":

> *The attack came with surprising ferocity. In a moment the nausea yielded to a chill that made Amporn feel her body was encased in a shroud of ice. Under the blazing tropical sun she shook uncontrollably. During this "freezing" rigor, Amporn's temperature had risen to 104°F. After an hour of tooth-chattering shakes the rigor abated and for a few moments in the eye of this parasitic storm Amporn thought she might yet live. The brief respite was followed by a feverishness that was as intense as the sensation of cold she had experienced during the rigor. Amporn's temperature was now 106°F. Her senses reeled; consciousness blurred. She crawled into her house and collapsed upon the cool dirt floor, her sarong sodden with the sweat pouring from her burning body.*

Ironically, it was the burning fever, so horrible a symptom of the disease, that convinced Viennese neurology professor Julius Wagner von Jauregg to inject people with the malaria protozoan. The year was 1917, and the seemingly insane idea was a new and revolutionary therapy for the treatment of late-stage syphilis. It was believed that the corkscrew-shaped heat-sensitive bacteria of syphilis would be killed by malaria-induced fevers. And it worked. A relatively harmless strain of malaria protozoan was injected into late-stage syphilis victims, those already showing signs of neurological damage. When the fever struck, it stopped the progression of the disease right in its tracks. People were not necessarily cured, but they got no worse. In this way tens of thousands of people were spared a certain, agonizing death, and in 1928 von Jauregg received a Nobel Prize for his insanity. Several years ago malaria therapy was even suggested for patients suffering Lyme disease, since it is caused by a spirochete very similar to the one responsible for syphilis. (For more on Lyme disease, see Chapter 5, "New Kids on the Block.")

The rigor, or shakes, so symptomatic of malaria is a consequence of the way the insidious malarial protozoan lives its life. It is a very complex life that involves both man and insect. It is, however, a life we must understand in intimate detail if we are to conquer this "mother of fevers," as the ancient Chinese called malaria.

Life cycle of a killer. To be precise, there are four species of the *Plasmodium* protozoan that infect humans and cause malaria, but one, *P. falciparum*, is particularly virulent and lethal. It accounts for over 95 percent of all malarial deaths. All four, however, have a similar life cycle.

Human infection begins with a bite from a female anopheles mosquito. Only anopheles mosquitoes are vectors of human malaria, and only females bite. The male, to quote Dr. Desowitz, "flies about in a lifelong pursuit of sex and nectar." (In many ways it is not unlike the human male.) With her bite the infected mosquito injects thousands of threadlike plasmodia called *sporozoites* into her victim. These sporozoites head straight for the liver, where each one infects a liver cell. In the liver cell the sporozoite rounds up and divides repeatedly, producing up to forty thousand spores. Spore production takes two weeks, during which time there are no signs of illness. But the seeds of malaria are being sown.

The first clinical attack—sweating and high fever—occurs when the liver cells burst, releasing their myriad spores into the bloodstream. Each spore invades a red blood cell within which it lives for a while, feeding on the cell's hemoglobin and growing large. Finally there is a shattering of the spore into smaller fragments—an asexual means of producing yet more spores (scientific name *merozoites*). When the red blood cell bursts, the merozoites are released and invade new blood cells. Repeated cycles of red blood cell infection and rupture ultimately lead to a chronic malarial condition or death.

There is an amazing synchrony to the invasion and bursting of red blood cells. For reasons not fully understood, it seems that millions of infected blood cells burst simultaneously, releasing their merozoites. It is this timed, en-masse slaughter of red blood cells that brings on a bout of the shakes.

After several rounds of blood cell infection and reinfection some of the merozoites get down and dirty, transforming into male or female reproductive cells—the *gametocytes*. This is where the human phase of the life cycle ends. When an anopheles mosquito sucks up malaria-infected blood, she also sucks up millions of gametocytes. In her stomach the gametocytes develop into eggs and sperms, and fertilization occurs.

In a final act of brilliance, the fertilized eggs grow into threadlike sporozoites and make their way to the salivary glands, completing the cycle (see Figure 1, Plasmodium Life Cycle). The mosquito is now a deadly vector of malaria.

Interestingly, the disease sickle-cell anemia and its milder form, sickle-cell trait, offer sufferers protection against malaria. They do this by deforming the red blood cells, thereby preventing the protozoa from flourishing within them. Small wonder sickle-cell is so common an inherited disease in highly malarious parts of the world.

Malaria kills more than a million African children each year. Perhaps another million die in South America and Asia. It is in these wet, tropical continents that the mosquitoes of malaria thrive. Surprisingly, however, throughout much of recorded history malaria was very much a European disease. Spreading northward from Africa, it invaded Greece and Italy in A.D. 79, devastating the very susceptible populations of these nations. The Roman Empire, so formidable in its day, was crippled by malaria. Roman soldiers carried the disease as far north as England and Denmark. For two millennia it plagued much of Europe, until its eradication in the late 1940s.

Malaria was a relative newcomer to the New World, not arriving there until Columbus and other European explorers brought their parasites with them to the Americas. But it did not take long for malaria to establish itself and become a serious endemic disease from southern Chile to Montreal. President George Washington suffered from malaria. So did Abraham Lin-

Figure 1 *Plasmodium Life Cycle*

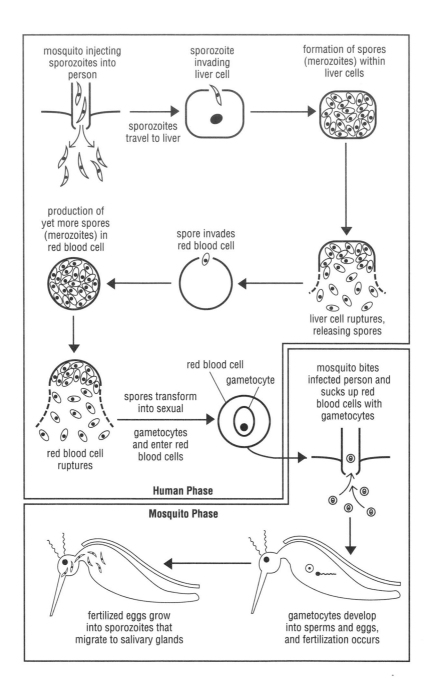

coln. During the Civil War half of the white troops and four-fifths of the African-American soldiers in the Union Army contracted malaria annually. Altogether at least a million soldiers suffered from malaria during the Civil War. In the 1930s, six hundred thousand Americans contracted malaria domestically. Atlanta, Georgia, was a hotbed of malaria, which was very much an American disease until about 1950, when eradication efforts wiped it out. From a unit created during World War II to control malaria, the CDC was born.

Prevention. How does one proceed to wipe out malaria? The most successful methods attacked not the protozoa but the mosquito. Eliminate their breeding sites, the standing water in which their young grow and develop, and you've eliminated the problem. Easier said than done. To quote a Tanzanian medical director, "These little creatures can breed thousands of offspring in a puddle the size of a hippo's foot."

Yet eliminate their breeding sites is exactly what Benito Mussolini did in the 1930s. Through elaborate canals he drained a region known as the Campagna, the wet, fertile area extending westward from Rome to the sea. It was, however, a monumental effort achieved at great expense. Such antimalarial endeavors were not even feasible for the rest of Italy, let alone the rest of the world. Obviously other methods of pest control were necessary and were employed with varying degrees of success.

A tried-and-true course of action for killing anopheles larvae (known as *wrigglers* because they wriggled in the water) was to lay down a film of oil on the breeding pools. The oil clogged larval breathing tubes, and the larvae died. Unfortunately, oiling had to be repeated quite often or mosquitoes returned.

Then it was noticed that young larvae pretty much swept any floating particle of the proper size into their mouths. Why not dust the water with a chemical that, upon ingestion, would kill the young anophelines? By about 1920 a suitable larvicide was found—Paris green. Cheap, effective, and noninjurious to other animals, it could even be broadcast over large, swampy areas by airplane.

At about the same time Paris green was being deployed in Italy and other European nations, a tiny fish of the genus *Gambusia* was generating excitement among malariologists. Native to North America, it demonstrated a voracious appetite for mosquito larvae. Why not ship gambusia to highly malarious countries, where it could be used to stock anopheles-infested waters?

Attacking anopheles at its water-dependent larval stage was not the only strategy employed against these malaria vectors. Before the turn of the nineteenth century, homes were often fumigated with smoke to kill adult mosquitoes. It was not easily done, however, and ruined much of the household furnishings. In 1910 an aqueous solution of pyrethrum, a powder derived from chrysanthemum flowers, was put into a spray bottle and became the first widely used insecticide. It worked very well in killing adult anopheles mosquitoes as well as other disease-carrying insects. In fact a 1944 epidemic of typhus, transmitted by a louse, was quelled by dusting the inhabitants of war-torn Naples, Italy, with pyrethrum. Regrettably, pyrethrum suffered the same shortcomings as those that had preceded it; namely, the insecticide had to be applied to surfaces at least once a week to be effective.

In their desperation to achieve some degree of success in combating malaria, scientists became remarkably inventive. One epidemiologist set up a ring of twenty pigsties around a malarious village, believing that the mosquito vectors would choose swine to feed on in lieu of humans. He even boasted some success, but like Paris green, oiling, and pyrethrum, it just didn't get the job done.

Then, in 1941, Paul Müller registered a new insecticide with the Swiss patent office—the office where Albert Einstein had worked while formulating his greatest theories. From this historic building would emerge patent no. 226150, the ultimate weapon against malaria—DDT. Dichloro-diphenyl-trichloroethane was everything anyone could ask for in an insecticide. It was inexpensive to manufacture. It appeared harmless to other animals, including humans. But most important, it killed all manner of insects and kept on killing. DDT was sprayed on walls, floors, and ceilings. Like pyrethrum, it was also dusted on people to kill the lice that spread typhus. But unlike pyrethrum, it had tremendous staying power. A DDT-treated surface would kill for up to six months. Needless to say, malariologists were ecstatic.

Early trials with DDT proved so successful that in 1947 the U.S. Congress appropriated $7 million for malaria eradication within its borders. By the early 1950s not one case of malaria could be found in America.

At long last eliminating malaria worldwide seemed more than just a dream. Malariologists predicted that massive and continued spraying in countries where malaria was endemic (most of the world) would completely stamp out the mosquito vector. Malaria would go the way of smallpox.

With such unbridled optimism WHO, backed mainly by U.S. dollars, embarked on a very ambitious five-year campaign to wipe malaria off the face of the planet. It began in 1958, and it almost worked. Malaria-ridden Sri Lanka, for example, went from one million cases in 1955 to just eighteen in 1963. Incidence of the disease was reduced dramatically in other countries as well.

The principal reason for DDT's failure to completely eradicate malaria was the anopheles mosquito's ability to develop resistance to the insecticide. Malariologists were experiencing what bacteriologists had encountered after the discovery of antibiotics. In time DDT-resistant populations of mosquitoes developed.

Growth of such resistant populations should have surprised no one. Individuals within a large population show varying degrees of DDT resistance. A select few might even be totally unaffected by the insecticide. Routine spraying would kill the vast majority of susceptible insects, leaving resistant survivors to go forth and multiply. To further complicate the issue, environmentalists began complaining that DDT was harming fish and fowl, demanding that its use be curtailed. Unfortunately, as soon as rigorous use of DDT was discontinued, the mosquitoes returned with a vengeance. Mortality due to malaria in 1993 was at a historic all-time high in Africa, and it is currently the only major disease other than AIDS and tuberculosis that is spreading steadily. A whopping 40 percent of the world's population is at risk for contracting malaria. And the returning plague seemed to be more lethal than ever. A new wrinkle had been added. A cerebral form of malaria had developed and was attacking the brain, killing people with alarming suddenness. What, if anything, could be done?

Treatment. Scientists did have one other weapon in their antimalarial arsenal—drugs with which to treat patients. Robert Koch, the brilliant microbiologist of tuberculosis fame, often said of malaria, "Treat the patient, not the mosquito." Unfortunately, in his day (late nineteenth century) there was only one drug—quinine.

Quinine, a preparation from the bark of the cinchona tree, had been used as an antimalarial for centuries by natives of South America. It was and still is an excellent antimalarial drug. Regrettably, however, it was and still is fairly toxic, often causing deafness when used in dosages necessary to kill plasmodium. Nonetheless, it was used universally and extensively until the 1930s, when other, less harmful derivatives were synthesized. Chief among them was chloroquine.

Shortly after its development chloroquine became the drug of choice for treating malaria. It would sit on the dinner table in stately homes alongside the salt and pepper shakers. Hospitals and the military handed out chloroquine as if it were candy. Undoubtedly chloroquine saved countless millions of lives through the 1940s and '50s, but its widespread, indiscriminate use would also be its undoing. By the early 1960s physicians around the world were beginning to report cases of malaria that would not respond to chloroquine. *Plasmodium falciparum* was evolving, adapting, becoming resistant to the drug. Soon drug-resistant malaria—not only to chloroquine but to other pharmaceuticals as well—became the rule rather than the exception. The magic bullet had lost its magic.

Today the search continues for drugs that will effectively halt *Plasmodium*. In July 2000 the FDA approved Glaxo Wellcome's Malarone for prevention and treatment of malaria. A synthetic drug called pyronaridine, developed in China, shows great promise. And there are others. Meanwhile, chloroquine has been largely replaced by mefloquine as the standard treatment for malaria. It is even recommended prophylactically for American travelers to Africa.

In retrospect the international effort to eradicate malaria might have been better served if conducted differently. Had all endemic areas been drenched with massive and repeated doses of DDT, had the entire tropical world been saturated simultaneously with chloroquine, the insect and/or its protozoan parasite might not have survived the onslaught. But that did not happen, and as soon as eradication efforts abated, the mosquito rebounded triumphantly.

Vaccination. By 1965 it became obvious to all concerned that the tag team of DDT and chloroquine was not going to snuff out malaria. WHO, looking for yet another magic bullet, turned its energies and financial resources to developing a vaccine. It had worked for Jenner and smallpox as well as a dozen other diseases. Why not malaria?

Why not? Because the malaria protozoan is vastly more complex than the viruses and bacteria that succumbed to vaccination. To begin with, plasmodium's life cycle involves at least six antigenically distinct types of organisms. Against which one should a vaccine be generated? And, unlike bacteria or viruses, scientists could not successfully grow and study plasmodium in a culture dish until 1977.

Nonetheless, grants were awarded liberally to any scientist with a laboratory, some anopheles mosquitoes, and a desire for a Nobel Prize. Soon vaccines began to appear. Some were made from infected red blood cells, ruptured and treated with formalin to attenuate the protozoa. Mosquitoes carrying plasmodium were irradiated with x-rays in hopes of beating their protozoa into a suitable vaccine. Plasmodium itself was grown in culture, and different concoctions of whole and fragmented protozoa were melded into vaccines. Yet by 1990 all attempts to provide effective immunity through vaccination had largely failed.

Then the big guns were brought in. The 1980s had seen major advances in molecular biology—advances such as DNA analysis, genetic engineering, improved methods of protein synthesis, and antibody production. With these powerful and sophisticated tools researchers prodded and poked poor plasmodium. By 1992 the first glimmer of hope appeared. Dr. Manuel Patarroyo of Colombia created a vaccine from proteins he had manufactured in the lab, proteins that were identical to those of the protozoan. Now, in effect, he had a synthetic parasite, or at least part of one, that could induce an immune response without causing disease. Trial tests conducted first in South America and later in Africa initially proved effective, reducing by nearly 40 percent the rate of infection in vaccinated subjects. In subsequent trials, however, the vaccine gave almost no protection against malaria to inoculated children. Back to the drawing board. Today we have anti-sporozoite vaccines and anti–asexual blood stage vaccines and transmission-blocking vaccines under investigation.

Meanwhile other scientists are picking apart the genes of anopheles and plasmodium, learning which ones produced resistance to DDT and chloroquine. Hopefully this knowledge can be used to make the deadly disease vulnerable once again to drugs and insecticides.

Is there yet hope for humanity in its quest to make the world malaria-free? Yes—but it won't come soon, it won't come easily, and it won't come cheaply. For the foreseeable future, the smart money is on the ingenuity and evolutionary prowess of *P. falciparum*.

Flatworms

Protozoa are not the only parasites that find humans particularly hospitable. Ticks, lice, and mites are other examples of parasites—external parasites, which feed on people without entering their bodies. Most important, however, as far as human disease and death are concerned, are two groups of internally parasitic worms. They are the flatworms and the roundworms, simple animals that have given up free-living for freeloading.

Tapeworm

Flatworms are the reason I do not eat steak tartare, for lurking in raw beef may be small, immature tapeworms. Fish and pigs are also carriers of tapeworm, so eating improperly cooked fish or pork is ill advised as well. Many Jewish people used to get tapeworm after eating a delicacy known as gefilte fish, prepared by boiling ground pike, carp, whiting, or other fish that has been seasoned and molded into balls. When gefilte fish is cooked insufficiently, tapeworm larvae can survive and find their way to the diner's digestive tract. There is even danger in preparing gefilte fish, for cooks have a tendency to taste-test the partially cooked fish as it simmers.

Tapeworms derive their name from the fact that the adult worm is long and ribbonlike—sometimes very long. That baby worm you accidentally ingest, once it attaches to your small-intestine wall (by means of hooks or suckers on its head), may grow to be sixty feet long (more than eighteen meters). And the worm is a very interesting creature in the way it conducts its life—the ultimate parasite, if you will. It has no mouth and no trace of a digestive system. They have been lost over time as the animal adapted to a way of life in which it merely soaks up digested nutrients like a sponge. What the tapeworm does possess is a highly developed reproductive system, for perpetuation of the species is the name of the game. It is hermaphroditic, and each individual worm has many testes and ovaries. Eggs are self-fertilized and then released in huge numbers with the feces. Some of these eggs will find a cow or pig to parasitize, and the life cycle of infection continues. Fish tapeworms follow a somewhat more circuitous route, first infecting tiny copepods, which are then eaten by the fish.

As with most parasites of the digestive system, proper sanitation and sewage disposal are essential to eradication of the disease. And, of course, thorough cooking of meat and fish will kill the larvae and prevent infection.

Tapeworms may make you weak, undernourished, and anemic. They can cause diarrhea and digestive system problems. In some instances the worm travels to other organs, leading to serious complications. When doctors autopsied one woman who had died of epileptic convulsions, they found her brain riddled with small encysted tapeworms. Usually, however, infection with these worms is not life-threatening or even particularly debilitating. Many times one becomes aware of tapeworm infestation only when part of the worm breaks off and is seen in the stool. Elimination of the worm involves taking drugs orally that literally put the worm to sleep. Only then will the head release its grip on the intestine wall and allow itself to be flushed out with a purgative. If the head is not removed, the worm simply grows back.

Tapeworms are certainly a nuisance and a potential danger. As agents of suffering and death, however, they pale in comparison to another class of parasitic flatworms, the flukes.

Schistosomiasis

Adult flukes are much smaller than tapeworms, but the devastation they cause is far greater. One type of fluke, the blood fluke or schistosome, is particularly nasty, causing a level of global debilitation by parasite that is second only to malaria. An estimated two hundred million people in seventy Asian, African, and South American countries harbor schistosomes. Three-quarters of a million will die this year. No one really knows, with any degree of accuracy, how many people suffer from schistosomiasis because the range of symptoms is so enormous. The worm weakens and kills in many unpleasant ways. Heart disease, epilepsy, kidney failure, cirrhosis of the liver, lung degeneration, and even cancer can result from infection with the blood fluke. It is an excruciating and debilitating disease affecting mostly school-age children.

Often the first sign of schistosomiasis occurs at puberty. A strange and scary thing happens—urine suddenly and inexplicably turns red with blood. So common is the event, signaling the onset of the disease, that among boys it has come to be considered a sort of male menstruation throughout much of Africa.

Bloody urine is a manifestation of the way in which the parasite conducts itself within its human host. Infection begins when a person, often a young child bathing or a farmer wading through his rice paddy, enters water polluted with tiny schistosome larvae. These tadpolelike critters, the size of pinheads, penetrate the skin, causing an initial and transient rash. Disappearance of the rash, however, does not indicate the end of infection. After a brief respite the worm enters the bloodstream and travels first to the liver, where it matures, and then to a vein. Here the schistosome takes up residence. The vein it chooses is a function of the schistosome species. One species heads for veins of the lower intestine. Another settles in the upper intestine. Yet a third kind makes its home in the veins surrounding the urinary bladder.

Male schistosomes are of a decent size, stout and about three-quarters of an inch long. The worm attaches to the vein's inner wall with two suckers on its head. Females, narrower and shorter, nestle themselves into grooves that run down the length of the male. Here they remain in monogamous conjugal bliss for the rest of their lives, which may be as long as thirty years. For most of those thirty years females will crank out an enormous number of eggs—about thirty-five hundred daily.

It is these eggs that are the chief source of pathogenicity in people. They do not remain harmlessly in the venous home of their parents but begin to burrow through the blood vessel. The eggs must make it to the interior of the bladder or intestine, where they will be discharged with the urine or feces. Only then can their life cycle continue, a life cycle that requires that they next parasitize a water snail. If there are no proper snails—and they have only a day to find one—the flukes cannot develop into the forms that will infect humans. The schistosomes will perish, and the chain of transmission will be broken. Unfortunately there are lots of snails in the feces-contaminated waters of the third-world tropics.

Many if not most of the eggs that leave the vein of their birth do not make it to the lumen of the intestine or bladder. Caught in the tissues of various organs, they bring about a cascade of immune system responses and overresponses. There is inflammation and swelling around the eggs. Abnormal tissue masses develop, and ultimately the symptoms of schistosomiasis set in.

At first glance, eradication of schistosomiasis does not seem to be insurmountable. There is no counterpart to the omnipresent malaria mosquito, whose bite is impossible to avoid. The solution in the case of schistosomiasis should be quite simple: stay out of snail-infested waters. Easier said than done. Rice farming is everywhere in southern Asia and Africa, and in the watery rice paddies snails abound. Merely add untreated human waste, with its untold numbers of schistosomes, and, presto, you have pain and suffering on a grand scale.

One human endeavor has even expanded—and greatly so—the mantle of the schistosome. It is the construction of dams to provide hydroelectric power for developing nations. Two of the most ambitious and most disastrous of these water impoundment projects were the Volta River Dam in Ghana and the Aswan High Dam in Egypt. Both created huge lakes of standing water hundreds of miles across with thousands of miles of shoreline. And both lakes became breeding grounds for the snails of schistosomiasis. In areas where the disease had been virtually unknown, infection has soared to over 90 percent of the population. So much for progress.

Robert Desowitz makes the point in his book *New Guinea Tapeworms and Jewish Grandmothers* that "if schistosomiasis were present in Sweden or the United States it would not be tolerated." The infection would be treated—we have drugs such as praziquantel that are effective against the fluke and not unduly toxic to humans. The vectors would be eliminated through molluscicides (snails are mollusks) and drainage programs. Proper treatment of sewage would destroy the fluke before it had a chance to infect any surviving snails. In short, measures would be taken to ensure the good health of the citizenry. Life is, indeed, cheaper in third-world countries.

Roundworms

When you buy a puppy or a kitten, standard veterinary procedure is to deworm the animal. A simple pill or two will do the trick. The parasites your young pet suffers from are roundworms, long threadlike creatures that can be seen wriggling about in the feces. In fact their scientific name, *nematode*, comes from the Greek word for "thread," *nema*. They are called *roundworms* because their bodies are not flattened as are those of tapeworms and flukes.

Roundworms are the most common and widespread of all parasites. No animal is without its roundworms; they even parasitize plants. Fifty-odd species of roundworms live within humans, a dozen of which are common parasites causing disease, disfigurement, and death. One in every four people suffers some kind of roundworm infection. As biological opportunists seeking to benefit at the expense of other organisms, roundworms have no peers.

Guinea Worm

The guinea worm has long been one of the more serious discomforts of the tropics. Only a decade ago in some villages, a quarter of the population was periodically incapacitated with fits of vomiting, diarrhea, and dizziness—all the result of the female guinea. Two to four feet long (the male is only an inch), she wanders through the body for a while before settling down just under the skin. Her appearance is that of a coiled varicose vein. But veins do not create blisters that discharge a milky fluid when submerged in water. The fluid contains thousands of larvae. Upon release they go on to infect a tiny crustacean called cyclops. It is the swallowing of larvae-laden cyclops that brings about human infection.

The guinea worm—known worldwide as the "fiery serpent"—most commonly attacks the legs, often causing painful inflammation and crippling muscle damage. Legs, however, are by no means the only sites of infection. As Dr. Donald Hopkins, an expert in tropical parasites, points out in the October 30, 1995, issue of *People* magazine: "I can show you pictures of a worm emerging from the back of a child's head. They come out of the chest and genitals. One once came out under a man's tongue. The swelling was so painful he couldn't swallow and he starved to death."

Native medicine men and even medical doctors would remove the worm by slowly and painfully winding it out onto a stick, perhaps a turn or two a day. In endemic regions it is not uncommon to see people walking with sticks taped to their legs around which worms are coiled. Evidence of worm infestation has been found in three-thousand-year-old mummies, and some speculate that the caduceus—symbol of the healing arts—is a visual representation of this ancient medical practice. If the procedure is not done properly, bacterial infection sets in and loss of a limb or death can result.

Recently there has been a serious and successful effort to wipe out the guinea worm through hygiene and water purification, which may involve the use of simple nylon swatch filters. A disease that a decade and a half ago afflicted 3.5 million people now debilitates a mere 25,000. It is anticipated that soon the guinea worm will become the second disease to be eliminated from the world (after smallpox)—and without "magic bullet" vaccines or medications.

Anisakiasis

What do they call sushi in New Orleans? Bait. Well, in Japan they call this preparation of sliced raw fish (and sashimi, a similar dish) a gastronomic delight. It is loved by millions of people who indulge their appetites daily. Unfortunately, several hundred Japanese diners pay dearly each year for their sushi and sashimi fondness. They contract anisakiasis.

Although not a serious worldwide problem in terms of numbers, the disease has spread to other countries, including the United States. Any lover of raw fish should be aware of the possible dangers involved. Often only hours after eating the fish, excruciating abdominal pain and vomiting of blood may occur. The one-and-a-half-inch larva of anisakis has been ingested along with the food and has buried its head in the inner stomach lining. A look through a gastroscope (a tube stuck down the throat and into the stomach) reveals an angry-looking, bloody ulcer two inches in diameter. At the center of the inflamed, craterlike wound, the worm's body, anchored by its head, undulates obscenely to and fro.

Sometimes the worm can be removed by pincers at the end of the gastroscope and no further medical intervention is required. At other times surgery of affected tissue is required. The worm larva may also attach to the small intestine wall farther down the digestive tract. When it does, symptoms of severe stabbing pain are not as immediate.

Hookworm

Thankfully, when one considers the sheer numbers of people that consume sushi and sashimi daily, infection with anisakis larvae is quite rare. This is not the case with hookworm, another intestinal roundworm parasite that is ubiquitous throughout much of the tropical and subtropical world.

The parasite is small—adults attain a length of about a half inch—and derives its name from the tiny hooks or plates within its mouth. These plates bite down onto the intestinal wall as the worm sucks in blood and tissue fluids. The outcome, if worms are numerous (several hundred or more), is severe, crippling anemia. It is the legacy of the disease. Infection as a child often results in physical and mental retardation.

As is the case with so many parasites, the worm is transmitted from one host to another through feces. Within the human waste are microscopic eggs that mature into tiny larvae when deposited into the soil. The hookworm larvae will then burrow through the skin of anyone walking barefoot. From there they enter the bloodstream and take an express trip to the intestine.

Interestingly, hookworm was a very serious problem in the United States until the latter half of the twentieth century. Wherever winters were mild and the soil did not freeze (which kills the worms) hookworm was endemic. Millions of people in the southern states were afflicted. The "barefoot boy with cheek of tan" often grew into the stereotypically lazy, shiftless, dull-witted southerner as a result of being bled from within by this insidious parasite. The scientific name, in fact, for one of the several common hookworm species is *Nectarus americanus*—"American killer."

Better sanitation and public health awareness and the wearing of shoes have minimized the problem in the United States. Worldwide, however, tens—perhaps hundreds—of millions of people still suffer from hookworm. Because symptoms of the illness are so easily misdiagnosed, one cannot even hazard a guess as to exact numbers. Estimates run as high as 25 percent of the planet's population, with sixty-five thousand dying each year. A 1980 World Bank study found that 85 percent of the residents of Java had hookworm. In these countries it continues to shorten life and greatly reduce its quality.

Filariasis

One cannot talk of crippling parasitic diseases without mention of the roundworms known as *filaria*. They are of great importance in western and central Africa, the Middle and Far East, and the New World from Mexico to Brazil. Of particular concern are two filarial worms that are close cousins. One causes river blindness and the other elephantiasis. Together they infect 140 million people.

Elephantiasis is the more dramatic of the two diseases. It derives its name from the immense swelling that is its most outstanding feature. Often the legs are involved, becoming so enlarged they resemble those of an elephant. Men's genitalia, when affected, assume gargantuan dimensions. One male elephantiasis sufferer could not walk unless he placed his testicles—the size of watermelons—in a wheelbarrow and carted them before him. Women's breasts may be similarly altered.

Such extreme swelling is the consequence of the female worm's reproductive activity. She is three to four inches long and lies in a lymph gland or duct, looking like coiled string. Each day she pumps out thousands of progeny in the form of tiny threadlike larvae called microfilaria. Over time the microfilaria clog lymph ducts, causing lymphatic fluid to collect and swell affected body parts.

It is through the bite of a mosquito known as *Culex* that the worm is spread from one human to another. *Culex*, ubiquitous throughout the tropics and subtropics, is particularly fond of filthy, stagnant water such as raw sewage. Not surprisingly, growth of large cities without proper sanitation has greatly increased its numbers. The filaria of elephantiasis was even introduced into the southern United States with African slaves but was eradicated by the 1920s.

When *Culex* sinks its little proboscis into a human, it sucks up, along with its blood meal, the microfilaria of elephantiasis. Within the mosquito the larvae continue to develop. Soon the insect is ready to bite again and transmit its parasite. This transmission can be halted by treating infected individuals once a year over a four- to six-year period with a single-dose combination of oral medicines. It is one of about a half dozen infectious diseases in the world considered to be completely eradicable. So is its filariasis twin—river blindness.

River blindness—endemic primarily in Africa—is transmitted by the blackfly, an insect that lives and breeds in fast-flowing streams and rivers rather than stagnant pools. Its bite introduces into the human host a species of filaria that is happiest when infiltrating the eyes and outer layers of the skin. It is here that thousands of the snakelike microfilaria can be found. A common outcome of ocular infection is impaired vision or blindness. (In a related disease, *Loa loa*, worms can actually be seen moving across the front of the eyeball.) People with skin parasites fare no better. The microfilaria cause disfiguring lesions, leading to ostracism. Itching can become so intense and unrelenting that it has driven some sufferers to suicide.

Amid all this human anguish are safe and effective antifilarial drugs. In the early 1980s the pharmaceutical giant Merck and Co. invented ivermectin, an antiparasite drug that works well against the filaria of river blindness, as well as elephantiasis. Several years later Merck donated the drug to needy nations (and continues to do so), where half a million people were already blind from the roundworms and a hundred million more were at risk. But the effort was a dismal failure. The health programs of these nations were so poorly run that ivermectin never made it to the people. Such are the difficulties in developing countries. In 1995 a second effort was initiated by the World Bank to treat the peoples of sixteen African nations where river blindness is most devastating. It met with limited success. Today philanthropic organizations such as the Carter Center have joined the endeavor, realizing that if 85 percent of the people in endemic regions are given a dose of ivermectin twice in one year the disease can be wiped out. It is a goal on which the Carter Center has put a 2007 target date.

Almost two billion people, a sizable fraction of Earth's inhabitants, suffer parasite infections. They kill; they maim; they make life unbearable. So prevalent are parasitic diarrheas that they have simply become a way of life. A doctor, upon examining the watery stool of his patient, asked how long it had been like that. With some surprise, the patient replied, "It's always been like that."

It doesn't have to be like that. Most of the serious parasitic diseases—malaria, kala-azar, schistosomiasis, filariasis—can be brought under control and in most cases eradicated. What it takes is determination and a serious commitment. Unfortunately in many cases neither the rich developed nations nor the governments of the affected nations themselves exhibit such commitment. And pharmaceutical companies will rarely do anything unless there is a profit. Where does that leave several billion people? Living with debilitating illness and dying young.

Parasitic Fungi: A Fungus Among Us

All life on this planet can be sorted into five kingdoms. The obvious ones are plants and animals. Flatworm and roundworm parasites discussed in this chapter belong to the animal kingdom.

With the invention and widespread use of the microscope, an unseen living world suddenly burst into view. It was the world of one-celled organisms. The larger unicellulars, those with a complex cell structure, were classified as protists. Protozoan pathogens are found in this kingdom. Bacteria, tiny, simple, and single-celled, comprise yet a fourth kingdom. They are life at its most fundamental. Viruses, inert particles of nucleic acid and protein, have no cellular structure and are not considered living entities. As such, they belong to no kingdom of living things.

There is, however, a fifth kingdom of life, one populated by organisms in which cells are uniquely fused into microscopic filaments and reproductive spores perpetuate the many different species. It is the kingdom *fungi*.

Most fungi are nonpathogenic, growing in the soil and feeding on its organic matter. Some derive sustenance from dead plant and animal remains. They are called *saprophytes*. A mushroom is a saprophytic fungus, as is the fuzzy green mold growing on your three-day-old strawberries. Some fungi, however, are parasitic, living on and feeding off the living. In the process they cause disease. We have all suffered at one time or another from a rash or infection of the skin as a result of a fungal invasion. Athlete's foot, jock itch, and ringworm are familiar examples.

Breathing in spores released by certain fungi can also cause illness. Most of the time it is due to allergic reaction and not infection. Mold spores are, after all, second only to dust mites as the most common indoor allergen. But in some people, usually those with enervated immunity, fungal spores can establish lung and then systemic infections. AIDS sufferers are constantly plagued by normally harmless fungi.

Being the consummate opportunists, fungi exploit any and every weakness in an individual. *Candida* is a perfect example. Every year *Candida*, a single-celled fungus better known as yeast, gives rise to twenty million cases of vaginal infection, primarily in women who are on antibiotic therapy. The antibiotics kill normal flora (bacteria) in the vaginal tract that keep yeast growth in check. The yeast then overrun the area. In babies,

Candida causes diaper rash and in the immunosuppressed, the mouth infection thrush.

Recently, another fungus has been implicated in a number of serious illnesses. It is *Stachybotrys*, a wet, greenish-black growth that the media have dubbed "killer mold." Is this merely hyperbole, or does *Stachybotrys* deserve its menacing moniker? No one really knows. In 1993 and 1994 acute pulmonary hemorrhage struck forty-seven infants living in the Cleveland, Ohio, area after homes had been flooded. Sixteen died. Since then sporadic cases have been reported. A CDC investigation concluded that significant exposure to *Stachybotrys* growing on and in the walls of many of the homes played a significant role in the development of this severe and oftentimes fatal lung disease. But other more common molds—aspergillus, penicillium, cladosporium—were also present and might have contributed to the problem.

Even if it is not the mass murderer portrayed in the tabloids, *Stachybotrys* does cause myriad symptoms that have come to be known as "sick building syndrome." These include coughing, wheezing, runny nose, eye irritation, sore throat, skin rash, diarrhea, headache, fatigue, and general malaise. Mycologist and *Stachybotrys* investigator Dr. Dorr Dearborn says, "it's like having a bad cold that doesn't go away." As with other fungi, *Stachybotrys* thrives in dark, wet places. Basements, especially those that take in groundwater or become very humid during warm weather, provide a perfect environment for *Stachybotrys*. Well-insulated, airtight buildings that do not "breathe" can exacerbate the situation. Studies have found the killer mold in 1 percent to 3 percent of homes tested. And as *Stachybotrys* grows it produces powerful toxins that can be found in its spores. Inhaling these poisonous spores in high enough concentration produces the flu-like symptoms of sick building syndrome or more serious lung disease.

Medical experts predict a dramatic rise in fungal infections as the population of weak and immunocompromised individuals in our society continues to increase. Nosocomials, those infections contracted in hospitals, will show the most striking upsurge with the old, sick, and weak being kept alive longer through the miracle of medicine. AIDS presents a frightening picture of how fungi can completely overwhelm the human body. Coccidiodes, a rare fungal lung infection, is found in 10 percent of AIDS sufferers. Thrush, the oral yeast infection with its patches of creamy white exudate overlaying a painful reddish inflammation, is one of the signature diseases of AIDS. But more on AIDS—acquired immunodeficiency syndrome—in the next chapter.

10

AIDS

When a person has sex, they're not just having it with that partner, they're having it with everybody that partner has had it with for the past ten years.

—OTIS RAY BROWN

Every once in a while a new disease will emerge and knock the socks off the human population. It happened with HIV/AIDS, and it can happen again.

—DR. ANTHONY FAUCI

A New Disease Emerges

In the fall of 1980 a very sick gay man entered the UCLA Medical Center. He was pale, very thin, had a mouth full of "cottage cheese," and coughed painfully and uncontrollably.

Examination revealed he had a fungal infection of the mouth called thrush and an exceedingly rare illness—*Pneumocystis carinii* pneumonia

(PCP)—caused by a protozoan. Doctors were baffled. Perhaps most puzzling was the complete absence of a certain population of white cells, called T4 cells, in the man's blood.

Pentamidine is a drug used to treat PCP, but PCP is so rare that hospital pharmacies do not stock it. Such "orphan drugs" that treat rare diseases and are considered experimental can be obtained only from the Centers for Disease Control and Prevention. UCLA doctors contacted the CDC and ordered the experimental drug for their dying patient. The CDC, in fact, had received five orders for pentamidine between September 1980 and May 1981—five orders in an eight-month period when they had received only two requests between 1967 and 1979. Clearly, something was amiss.

In July 1981 a man with purplish blue splotches covering his body entered San Francisco's General Hospital. He was a homosexual prostitute, and he had an extremely rare cancer. Called Kaposi's sarcoma (KS), it affected the blood vessels of the skin, causing out-of-control growth. At about the same time a cluster of KS cases occurred in New York City and Los Angeles as well.

By the end of August 1981 the CDC would report 107 cases of either KS or PCP or a combination of the two. AIDS had emerged, and in the ensuing two decades would create an unprecedented public health crisis. Medicine would marshal its forces as never before to wage war against a disease that has threatened to become the worst plague ever to afflict humankind. Through the 1990s, it was the leading killer of Americans aged twenty-three to forty-four. In 2000 it newly infected more than three million people. Year 2001 saw more people diagnosed with HIV infection in England than ever before, and Britain's Public Health Laboratory Service expects the number of cases to reach thirty-four thousand by 2005, a jump of 47 percent from 2000. As 2001 drew to a close, about twenty-two million people had died of AIDS worldwide, with another forty million infected, most asymptomatically. Nearly one million of them reside in the United States. The devastation it has wrought in Africa, where 70 percent of cases occur, is not to be believed. AIDS kills three times as many people in Africa as the next most common cause of death. In eleven million people it has also teamed up with the bacillus of tuberculosis, making TB many times more deadly (see Chapter 4, "The White Death"). The life expectancy of a child in Botswana has dropped from seventy years to under forty as a result of AIDS.

The AIDS virus presently kills three million people annually, and by the year 2020 will have caused more fatalities than any other disease outbreak in history, including the Black Death of the fourteenth century, which mowed down one-third of Europe's population. Some extrapolations put the figure of those infected at one billion by the year 2050. That's one out of every six people.

Thankfully, however, onset of the disease is no longer a death sentence. At one time AIDS, along with rabies, was considered the most lethal of all viral infections, with mortality figures at or very near 100 percent. Advances, however, in treatment of both AIDS and its many opportunistic infections have greatly extended life expectancies.

In the beginning AIDS was primarily, if not solely, found among homosexual males. And its most distinguishing feature was a total collapse of the immune system. Hence the disease's original designation, *gay-related immune deficiency—GRID*.

Annihilation of the immune system in AIDS is accomplished by selective destruction of one key class of white blood cells—the helper Ts or T4 cells. As discussed earlier (see Chapter 6, "The Virus"), T4 cells are a central player in any immune response. Simply put, they release chemicals called *interleukins* that turn on every other component of the immune system. Destroy them, and the entire immune response goes kaput.

With no system to fight invading microorganisms, the body is prey to any number of weird and highly unusual diseases. Known as *opportunistic infections*, they are caused by germs that exploit a decimated immune system to gain biological advantage within our bodies. The two most common and devastating opportunistic infections are *Pneumocystis carinii* pneumonia and Kaposi's sarcoma. Together they have become the signature of AIDS. But many other odd ailments make the life of an AIDS sufferer a veritable hell. Diseases formerly found only in sheep, cats, or birds suddenly appear in AIDS patients. Laurie Garrett, in her tome *The Coming Plague*, lists the more important ones:

> *Thrush caused by* Candida *fungal infections; pronounced* herpes simplex-II *throughout the body; blood contamination of active*

cytomegalovirus *with unknown effect; mononucleosis due to* Epstein-Barr *virus; marked lymph node swelling; radical infections of the stomach and gastrointestinal tract with* Entamoeba histolytica; *diarrhea and gastric problems caused by the* Cryptosporidium *parasite; similar symptoms caused by, of all things,* Mycobacterium avium, *a tuberculosis bacteria usually found in chickens; galloping infections in many organs of the* Cryptococcus *fungus; out of control bacterial infections with common organisms such as* Staphylococcus aureus, Escherichia coli *and* Klebsiella.

What on earth could so devastate an immune system? Was it a deadly chemical? Was it an infectious agent? Was it the wrath of God descending on homosexual sinners, as certain evangelists claimed? A frantic search for the cause of AIDS began.

Searching for the Cause

It was apparent from the outset that AIDS was preferentially attacking gay men. What was it, epidemiologists wanted to know, that singled them out? One common factor among all the initial cases of 1980 and early 1981 was a promiscuous lifestyle. Ever since the 1969 Stonewall riots in Greenwich Village—when police tried to shut down a gay bar called Stonewall and arrest its patrons—the gay community had "come out of the closet." Homosexuals began demonstrating, becoming vocal and politically active in their demands for equal rights. Gay bathhouses opened up that were nothing short of orgy centers. This sudden sense of freedom caused a small but significant group of gay men to overindulge in casual sex. For some men that meant as many as several hundred partners a year!

It was predominantly this population that was contracting AIDS. With promiscuity as a common thread, researchers came up with various and sundry theories to account for its transmission. Ideas ranged widely. One leading theory proposed that sperm of a sexual partner was finding its way into a victim's bloodstream. His immune system then made antibodies to the sperm that cross-reacted with his own T cells. What was, in effect, happening was an autoimmune response triggered by foreign sperm. But why would sperm suddenly start turning deadly?

Another popular misconception was that amyl nitrite, known as "poppers," was causing the symptoms. Used to intensify orgasms during sexual encounters, amyl nitrite also suppresses the immune system. There was no reason, however, to ascribe sustained and continued immune system collapse to poppers taken months earlier. More and more, GRID was exhibiting the transmission characteristics of an infectious, sexually transmitted disease. But what infectious agent was being transmitted?

At first the notion of "antigen overload" was promulgated by some researchers. They suggested that rather than a single germ causing GRID, a host of sexually transmitted viruses and bacteria were battering the immune system over the years, seriously overworking and depleting the T-cell population. However plausible and seductive the overload theory appeared to some investigators, it could not explain why, in the summer of 1982, hemophiliacs began developing GRID. Couple that with the appearance of GRID among intravenous drug addicts and people receiving blood transfusions, and it became clear that the disease was blood-borne—spread by some mysterious infectious agent in the blood. No longer a strictly homosexual affliction, the disease was renamed AIDS—acquired immune deficiency syndrome—in late 1982. Could it be that the wrath of God was now bearing down on innocent heterosexuals?

AIDS was an infectious, blood-borne disease that could also be transmitted sexually. Soon the mad pursuit began, with labs around the globe racing one another to isolate the bug that gobbled up T cells. Its discovery would certainly mean fame, fortune, and a Nobel Prize.

One scientist whose curiosity was piqued by the notion of an infectious agent, probably a virus because it was so hard to detect, was Robert Gallo. It was the involvement of T cells that most intrigued him. A few years earlier he had shocked the scientific establishment by announcing the discovery of a new and highly unique human virus that infected T cells, turning them cancerous. The virus was dubbed *HTLV*, named after the disease it caused—human T-cell leukemia. HTLV was the first human retrovirus ever isolated.

A retrovirus is a very special entity. Like many other viruses, it has RNA as its genetic material. But unlike other viruses, the RNA does not directly synthesize protein. First it goes in reverse, making DNA. The DNA then makes another RNA strand that finally goes about manufacturing protein (see Chapter 6, "The Virus").

Why such needless nucleic acid synthesis? It is analogous to your taking a perfectly fine loaf of bread back to the store and exchanging it for a new loaf before making a sandwich. What a monumental waste of time and energy for both you and the virus. Or is it? Rarely do living systems evolve mechanisms that do not in some way benefit the organism, and retroviruses are no exception. The apparent senseless production of unnecessary DNA is of great benefit to the virus, for it allows it to incorporate itself into the host cell's DNA. In a process called *integration* the viral DNA splices itself right into the host's genome.

Integration, a process essential and unique to retroviral replication, affords the virus several distinct advantages. First, the virus, now part of the host genome, is well hidden from detection and destruction by the ever-vigilant immune system. Second, with each cell division the virus—or, more precisely, the viral DNA—replicates and goes into a new cell. Silently the virus spreads throughout the organism. And if infection happens to occur in gamete-producing cells of a testis or ovary, sperms and eggs might even carry the internalized virus to the host's offspring.

Although many if not most retroviruses probably travel within host cells causing little or no harm, sometimes integration alters the cell in such a manner as to turn it malignant. This is the type of retrovirus—HTLV—that Robert Gallo discovered in 1979. In 1982 his lab isolated a second, closely related T-cell leukemia virus, which he named *HTLV-2* (the first became *HTLV-1*).

Could AIDS, Gallo speculated, also be caused by a retrovirus? And if so, was it one of the HTLVs, or was it a totally new virus? Both HTLV and the AIDS virus infected T cells and suppressed the immune system. Both were transmitted through blood and sex. This was compelling evidence.

By mid-1982 Gallo's lab initiated investigations to find the AIDS virus. Step one was to determine whether or not it was a retrovirus. This could be accomplished by growing the virus in cell culture and testing for retroviral activity. All retroviruses have a unique enzyme that allows them to churn out DNA from an RNA template. The enzyme is found only in retroviruses—their footprint, if you will—and demonstration of its presence in cell cultures is clear proof of retroviral infection.

The only problem, in early investigations, was the near impossibility of getting enough virus to grow in culture. The reason was simple. Unlike

HTLV, which caused T4 cells to grow and multiply indefinitely (as cancerous cells are wont to do), the AIDS virus seemed to destroy the T cells they replicated within. Not until late 1983 was a T-cell line found that could maintain the suspected AIDS virus without itself being destroyed. Now the AIDS virus could be grown in abundance.

With this new batch of T cells and AIDS-infected tissues, Gallo and his team of virologists went about testing for retroviral activity. When they found it, they tested for the presence of HTLV. This was done by mixing the infected samples with antibodies to HTLV. A reaction meant that the virus was most likely present in the tissues. At this point an even more conclusive test for HTLV presence was performed in which DNA probes for HTLV were used. Bonding of the probe with DNA in the AIDS tissues would indicate the presence of HTLV.

By April or May of 1984, after many months of growing and testing and learning how to handle the cultures, success was realized. A new virus had been found. It demonstrated the enzymatic activity of a retrovirus but did not react with antibodies to HTLV-1 or HTLV-2. Most important, it was found in a substantial number of AIDS patients and people at risk for AIDS. No evidence of the virus was found in 115 healthy heterosexuals. Robert Gallo named the virus *HTLV-3* and declared it to be the infectious agent that produced AIDS.

As it turned out, Gallo was correct. HTLV-3 was the cause of AIDS. He was not, however, the first to discover it. That honor went to Luc Montagnier of the Pasteur Institute in France. A year earlier he had isolated a retrovirus from a section of swollen lymph node excised from an early-stage AIDS patient. But when he published his findings, claiming it to be the AIDS virus, the scientific community did not feel he had proven his case.

What ensued was a bitter and ugly battle between Gallo's National Cancer Institute (part of the National Institutes of Health [NIH]) and Montagnier's Pasteur Institute. Both demanded credit for discovery of the virus. Things really heated up when the DNA of each virus was sequenced and the two were compared. The match (nearly 99 percent) was so perfect between the two that they could only have come from the same patient.

The implications were enormous. Both labs, during the course of their investigations, had exchanged tissue samples as well as other reagents—antibodies, cell culture growth factors, and the like. Had Gallo taken Montagnier's virus and deliberately tried to pass it off as his own independently isolated one? Had Montagnier's virus mistakenly contaminated Gallo's cultures, making its isolation an unfortunate but innocent laboratory error? No one would ever know for certain, but in March 1987 the governments of France and the United States intervened to call an armistice between the feuding labs. An agreement was announced officially recognizing the Montagnier and Gallo groups as codiscoverers of the AIDS virus, which was now being called *human immunodeficiency virus—HIV.*

The March 1987 accord also settled another long-standing dispute concerning patent rights to an AIDS blood test that had been developed in 1984. Gallo's group first developed the test, but Montagnier claimed that he did so using the Pasteur Institute virus. At first the U.S. Patent and Trademark Office awarded patent rights to Gallo, only to reverse its decision later on. The awarding of these rights was by no means academic since it would generate huge sums of money as blood tests were sold and used worldwide.

Financial gain notwithstanding, President Ronald Reagan of the United States and Prime Minister Jacques Chirac of France agreed to include the names of both Gallo and Montagnier on any and all blood test patents. Any royalties that accrued would go toward funding future AIDS research. Cooler heads had finally prevailed.

Testing for AIDS

By mid-1984 Gallo had finally found his AIDS virus. That was also an election year for President Reagan—a president who had been accused by many of being indifferent to the plight of AIDS sufferers. The last thing Reagan wanted to deal with was a tainted blood supply. So in June of 1984 five pharmaceutical companies were given twenty-five liters of T4 white cells infected with Gallo's HTLV-3 AIDS virus. Each was instructed to develop a reliable, economical blood test for HIV infection that could be performed quickly and easily.

Right from the outset all five companies realized that a practical, easily performed test must search not for the hard-to-detect virus but for antibodies to the virus circulating in the blood. A technique was employed called the *enzyme-linked immunosorbent assay*, or *ELISA* for short.

Today ELISA is still the most commonly used AIDS test for initial blood screening. It works something like this:

Small containers are provided by the pharmaceutical company. The walls of each container are impregnated with HIV antigens—the viral proteins that evoke strong antibody production during infection. Blood being tested is placed in the container and then washed out. Any antibodies to HIV present in the blood will cling to the antigens on the wall. Antibodies, however, are not visible. To determine whether any have stuck to the antigen layer, another chemical—chemical A—which binds to HIV antibodies, must be added. If HIV antibodies are present, chemical A forms a third layer that will not be washed off. Chemical A also has an enzyme attached to it that will make yet another chemical—chemical B—turn color. So a color change when chemical B is finally added indicates the presence of HIV antibodies and a positive test result for HIV infection. The procedure is summarized in Figure 2.

ELISA is a very reliable test, but it is not foolproof. Sometimes it does produce false positives. To make certain the positives are genuine, a backup test is needed. The most common confirmatory procedure is the Western Blot.

Like ELISA, the Western Blot tests for HIV antibodies in the blood. But it uses a wider range of viral proteins, derived from mashed-up viruses that have been separated from one another and fixed onto a solid strip of nitrocellulose. The result is greater sensitivity and accuracy in picking up HIV antibodies when the strip is washed with infected blood. One other minor difference between the two procedures is use of a radioactive chemical in the Western Blot to recognize HIV antibodies adhering to the strip. The radioactivity is detected by placing the strip onto a photographic plate.

Sometimes the roles of antigen and antibody are reversed, and the initial "solid" layer is of HIV antibodies and not viral antigens. When washed with blood, viruses themselves will adhere to the test strip or container. The great advantage of this test is that it detects infection very early, before the person begins developing antibodies.

Early detection of HIV infection is critical. It is for this reason that researchers adopted a state-of-the-art viral identification procedure called PCR analysis from the forensic lab. PCR (polymerase chain reaction) made headlines during the 1995 murder trial of O. J. Simpson. The test was used

Figure 2 *ELISA Test*

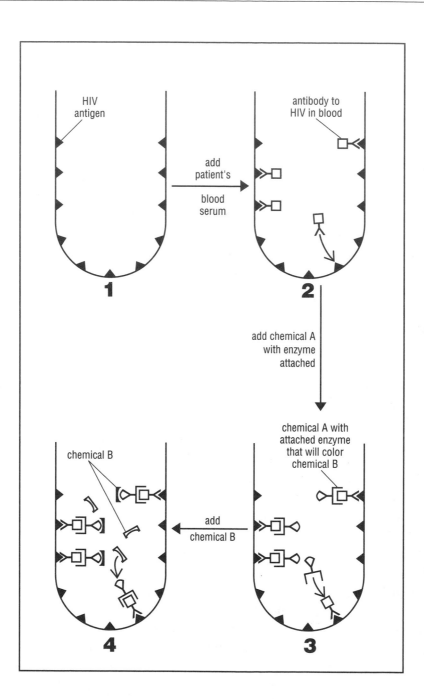

to compare DNA from blood at the crime scene with that of Mr. Simpson. That is what PCR does. It takes minuscule amounts of DNA and, using special enzymes, makes millions of exact copies until there is enough to study and test. In the case of HIV the procedure is able to hunt down the tiniest amounts of virus present within infected cells long before symptoms of the disease or even detectable antibodies appear.

Through the use of PCR researchers made a startling discovery. People can be infected with HIV for years before their blood tests positive for HIV antibodies—years in which they are unwittingly contagious. When it comes to viral infection, it seems that HIV breaks all the rules. The more we learn about the virus, the more it confounds us. And we have learned an awful lot in a relatively short period of time.

Without doubt HIV has become the most intensively studied virus in history. Scientists have dissected its proteins and mapped its genes. They have studied its every move as it performs its most dastardly intracellular deeds. What have we learned?

Anatomy of a Virus

In the spring of 1985, U.S. Secretary of Health and Human Services Margaret Heckler announced the discovery of a new retrovirus as the cause of AIDS. According to Ann Giudici Fettner in her book *The Science of Viruses*, an immunology researcher she was sitting with at the time blanched and groaned. "Oh God," he said, "we're in big trouble."

His words were prophetic to say the least. Although Ms. Heckler predicted a vaccine in five years, it is now seventeen years since her speech, and no vaccine is in sight. Some researchers wonder if an effective prophylactic vaccine can ever be created given the nature of HIV. It is like no other virus.

The outer, fatty envelope of HIV is actually a snippet of cell membrane that it steals and cloaks itself with as it exits a cell. Protruding from the fatty or lipid membrane, like so many warts on a toad's back, are knoblike projections of a sugary protein called glycoprotein 120 (gp 120). A second type of glycoprotein—gp 41—is embedded in the viral envelope and anchors the gp 120. These substances have been the subject of much research since they are the structures that first recognize and bind the virus to its target cells.

Beneath the lipid layer is a matrix layer of protein that surrounds the viral core. The core is the guts of the virus, where the nucleic acid resides in the form of two single RNA strands. These RNA strands house nine genes that code for fourteen different proteins. Joining the RNA within the core are several important enzymes that are needed to initiate infection.

By viral standards HIV is not particularly large or complex (although it is more complex than most other retroviruses). The smallpox virus is many times larger and contains enough DNA to control production of two hundred to three hundred proteins. Compare that to HIV's paltry nine genes coding for fourteen viral proteins. Yet finding a vaccine against small-pox was child's play compared to HIV. As Mark Caldwell so aptly put it in his August 1993 *Discover* article on AIDS, "Smallpox stumbles into the immune system like some dim-witted thug, setting off alarms everywhere." In 1796 Edward Jenner, not even aware of the existence of viruses, was able to scare up a smallpox vaccine from the pus of a milkmaid's cowpox sores. Why, by contrast, is HIV so impossibly difficult to battle?

In a word, stealth. HIV is no dim-witted thug, but rather a highly prac-ticed and skilled cat burglar. Action begins when viruses enter the body through tainted blood or, as is the most common route today, through unprotected sex. AIDS is sexually transmitted by virtue of the fact that the semen of an infected male is loaded with T4 white blood cells, which are, in turn, teeming with HIV.

Once introduced into the vagina or anus of a sexual partner, HIV and HIV-infected cells make their way into the bloodstream via tiny cracks in the mucous membrane. Here the virus encounters T4 cells, which are the primary targets of HIV. Sitting on the surface of T4 cells are proteins called CD4 markers. It is, in fact, the CD4 surface protein that gives the helper T its name—T4. These CD4s fit hand-in-glove with the gp 120 viral pro-jections. Using its gp 120s, the virus docks on the cell surface. Then, through a mechanism employing the other surface glycoprotein, gp 41, fusion of HIV's lipid coat with the cell membrane takes place. This is how HIV gains entry into the T4 cell, opening up and spilling its guts into the cell's interior.

Once inside the cell, HIV, being a retrovirus, uses its two single strands of RNA and the enzyme attached to them—reverse transcriptase—to make double-stranded DNA. It then integrates that DNA into the host's genome.

Although T4 cells are the primary targets of HIV, they are not the only ones infected. There is evidence that certain cells of the mucous membrane are also cloaked with CD4 markers. So cells susceptible to HIV infection probably line the vagina and anus. What more could a sexually transmitted virus ask for?

What more? How about the ability to infect macrophages? These, you may remember, are the large white blood cells that roam the body, swallowing up invading germs. Once inside macrophages, HIV get a free ride anywhere they want to go. It is believed that macrophages carry the viruses across the blood-brain barrier to the brain, where they bring about the dementia so common in advanced AIDS cases.

Many doctors and researchers feel that once integration occurs, there is little anyone can do to wipe the infection completely from the body. The immune system will not recognize and destroy cells that have HIV nestled snugly and safely within their nuclei. In effect, the body does not fight these viruses because these viruses have become part of the body.

Please do not, however, misunderstand what takes place during HIV infection. The virus does not remain quiescent for years as was originally thought. From the time a person first acquires HIV, many T4 cells begin actively replicating viral particles, and there is a vigorous initial immune defense. Large numbers of viruses are present in the bloodstream during this acute phase, and the patient experiences flulike symptoms for several weeks. Soon B cells start churning out antibodies to neutralize viruses not within cells, and activated killer Ts (see Chapter 6, "The Virus") destroy those cells already infected.

This brings the infection under control, but a fierce struggle between immune system and virus persists throughout the asymptomatic period of the disease—which typically lasts eight or nine years. Hundreds of millions of HIV are killed daily. At the same time the immune system can lose up to a billion T cells a day. During this period of stalemate between the virus and the immune system, the victim is said to be HIV-positive but does not yet suffer from AIDS. Slowly, however, over the years, the battle turns in favor of the virus. The invading hordes of HIV eventually overpower the huge and efficient armies of killer T cells and antibodies. Success is primarily a function of the virus's extreme mutability. Of all known viruses HIV has, by far, the highest rate of mutation. The same virus, over the course of infection in a single individual, can change its genetic makeup by as much as 30 percent. This is incredible variability—much more so even than the highly mutable influenza virus.

The reason for such genetic instability is the imprecise way in which reverse transcriptase makes DNA from viral RNA. In short, it makes mistakes, many of them, during transcription. And the high rate of viral replication, perhaps a billion new viral particles a day, only gives HIV more opportunity to mutate. Although most mutations hurt the virus and make it nonfunctional, every so often a mutant particle might arise with a slightly different surface protein—one that the immune system cannot recognize. Now a new population of viruses can run amok until the immune system catches up. Eventually so many mutants are generated that the immune army starts chasing its own tail, and the battle is lost.

Interestingly, much of the head-to-head combat between virus and T cell goes unnoticed because it occurs in the dozens of lymph nodes found throughout the body, not in circulating T4s. Lymph nodes are a part of our immune system, a filtering system of sorts that catches and destroys invading microbes. It now seems that T4 cells residing in lymph nodes are sitting ducks for HIV. During much of the asymptomatic period of AIDS infection, the viral load continues to build in these nodes. Meanwhile the T4 count in the bloodstream does not diminish appreciably. Finally the nodes "burn out," and virus floods into the blood, signaling the onset of full-blown AIDS. It is at this point that doctors, monitoring the blood, begin to notice a significant drop in levels of circulating T4 cells.

Nasty little critters, these HIVs. Can anything be done to stop them or even slow them down? Yes, but the task is a daunting one.

Prevention

Most experts agree that the global AIDS pandemic can be stopped only through an effective vaccine. The principle behind vaccination is remarkably simple. Present a harmless version of the germ to the immune system, and it will be duped into a state of readiness. Should the genuine article come along, it will be dealt with swiftly and harshly.

Such approaches have worked well with other viral diseases such as smallpox, polio, measles, and influenza. Either attenuated or killed viruses may be used. Attenuated virus seems to elicit better immune responses and is the vaccine of choice when feasible.

Concerning HIV, however, scientists are very reluctant to inject healthy people with weakened yet live virus. There is too great a danger that HIV will mutate to a not-so-weak form. Researchers dare not use even a killed vaccine for fear that some viral particles may have survived the killing process. One solitary surviving particle can invade a cell and initiate a cycle of infection.

Even if an attenuated HIV does not revert to virulence, there is always the possibility that it can reacquire the ability to integrate into the host genome. No one knows what long-term effect integrated HIV might have on a cell. With other human retroviruses it often leads to cancer. The last thing researchers want is a vaccine that will prevent AIDS only to produce a malignancy ten or fifteen years down the road.

For this reason there are no candidate live-attenuated HIV or whole-killed HIV vaccines in any human clinical trials. So where does that leave researchers? The only option is the creation of vaccines from harmless pieces, or subunits, of the virus. Up until recently, the focus has been on the envelope glycoproteins gp 120 and gp 41. They were the logical choice because they initiate infection, are easily accessible to antibodies, and do seem to elicit strong antibody production. Early vaccination attempts offered only short-lived and limited immunity, as mutability of the virus, once again, reared its ugly head. It is hard to find a magic bullet when the target keeps zigzagging every which way. A subunit vaccine can induce antibody production against only one type of subunit. If an HIV changes its subunit sufficiently, antibodies generated against the vaccine will not recognize it, and there will be no immunity.

This notwithstanding, the AIDS vaccine furthest along in the clinical testing process is of the subunit class. Called AIDSVAX, it is the first vaccine to enter Phase III trials—the final stage of testing—in which the effectiveness of the product is evaluated in large numbers of humans. Phase I and Phase II clinical testing deals primarily with safety issues.

A more recent vaccination strategy, the "naked DNA" vaccine, seeks to confer protection by using the actual genes of HIV. Once introduced into the skin or muscle, the genetic material is taken up by cells of the body, which then produce HIV proteins that stimulate the immune system.

Experimental vaccines using SIV (simian immunodeficiency virus) genes to protect monkeys against their form of AIDS have proved successful and Phase I trials with HIV genes are underway now in humans.

Genes of HIV need not, of course, be injected as naked bits of DNA. They can be inserted into a harmless virus or bacterium and then introduced into the body via this microbial vector. Once in the body, HIV genes will begin to express themselves and produce HIV proteins to which the immune system will respond. The concept is not new. Bacteria molecularly engineered to contain human insulin or growth hormone genes have been pumping out these hormones for more than twenty years.

In the eighteenth century, Edward Jenner discovered that immunization with cowpox protected people against variola virus, the cause of smallpox in humans (see Chapter 2, "Germs and Disease: A Brief History"). This concept of "Jennerian" vaccines, based on the use of similar but not identical viruses to those that cause disease, is being considered for HIV. Although not in clinical trials yet, possibilities include the simian equivalent of HIV (SIV) and a weaker strain of HIV called HIV-2.

Because of the extreme difficulty in trying to mount an immune assault against the wily, ever-metamorphosing HIV, efforts are being made to create a vaccine that directs immune responses against the human host cell receptors that serve as HIV's port of entry into cells. By blocking HIV receptors such as CD4, the virus will be unable to attach to the cell surface, preventing infection. It is a clever and novel approach and one that still awaits clinical testing.

With so many irons in the fire, one would hope that an AIDS vaccine is close at hand. But vaccine research is painstakingly slow. Clinical trials seem to take forever and often fail to produce the desired results. What appears so promising in a test tube or an experimental animal can fail miserably in human testing. The bottom line is that prospects for an effective, reliable prophylactic vaccine in the near future remain dim. Researchers feel that we'll be lucky to have even a crude one on the market by 2007. At current rates of infection, an additional fifty to one hundred million people will have contracted the virus by then, and millions will have died. In light of this, virologists and immunologists are working feverishly to find antiviral drugs that can stop or at least slow HIV infection. Since 1987 the drug of choice has been AZT.

Treatment

AZT, also known as azidothymidine, zidovudine, and retrovir, is one of a class of compounds dubbed nucleoside analogs, or nukes. Others include abacavir, 3TC, ddC, ddI, and D4T (the longer scientific names are not important). All are molecules that very much resemble one of the subunits—nucleosides—that are strung together by reverse transcriptase to make retroviral DNA. They are, in fact, DNA building blocks. What AZT and the other nukes do is fool the transcriptase into using them instead of the proper nucleoside. Proper nucleosides have a chemical hook on either end. One hook attaches to the growing DNA strand, while the other allows additional nucleosides to be attached. With nukes there is only one hook. Once the nuke is in place along the DNA chain, growth of the chain terminates and viral replication is halted.

There is another class of drugs that also cripple the functioning of reverse transcriptase. They are not, however, nucleoside analogs, hence the term *non-nucleoside reverse transcriptase inhibitors* (*NNRTIs*), and their mode of action is entirely different from the nukes.

Unfortunately, in a matter of months variants of reverse transcriptase appear in HIV that can produce viral DNA in the presence of either variety of inhibitor. Add to this the high toxicity level of nukes—up to 40 percent of the people on AZT are unable to tolerate it for more than six weeks due to the severe anemia it causes—and they are far from the ideal drugs.

The thought then crossed the minds of AIDS researchers to use two or even three nukes simultaneously, forcing the virus to undergo many more mutations to become resistant to the combination. Such double and triple drug therapies have indeed proved more effective than AZT alone and should buy more time for the AIDS sufferer. They are not, however, the knockout punch scientists are looking for. HIV will not succumb to one or even a combination of drugs aimed at a single step in its life cycle.

Which brings us to protease inhibitors (PIs)—another important weapon in our battle with HIV. Protease is one of the enzymes that HIV carries in its core. During the latter stages of viral infection protease is called on to perform a necessary step in synthesis of intact viral particles. It acts as a molecular scissors, snipping long protein molecules into smaller functional units. If this is not done, the virus cannot be assembled properly.

Scientists, of course, would like nothing more than to keep HIV from assembling properly. Toward this end they have come up with drugs that interfere with protease action—gum up the scissors, if you will. They are the protease inhibitors.

Serious testing of protease inhibitors began in 1995, with much scientific fanfare and unbridled optimism. To begin with, PIs were much less toxic than AZT and other nukes. And initial studies showed that they brought about almost complete cessation of viral replication. But, as with AZT, the protease inhibitors must deal with HIV's incredible ability to alter itself and its proteases so inhibitors will no longer inhibit. This explains the rationale behind combination drug therapy—the prescribing of one or more nukes in conjunction with protease inhibitors. To quote Dr. David Ho, head of New York's Aaron Diamond AIDS Research Center: "With protease there's been virtually a 98 to 99 percent inhibition of the virus. That's pretty potent. Add another drug like that, or a third one, and you start to pile them up, and just think about the kind of pressure that you put on the virus" (*New York Magazine*, February 20, 1995).

These AIDS "cocktails"—formally known as *highly active antiretroviral therapy (HAART)*—are a grueling regimen of strictly scheduled pill popping. Add to that the antivirals and antibacterials needed to control opportunistic infections, and the number of capsules climbs to as many as two dozen a day. But they are strikingly effective, and by 1997 had substantially reduced the number of AIDS deaths in the United States and Europe. It is lamentable that, at upwards of fifteen thousand dollars a person per annum, the treatments were largely unavailable to the millions of afflicted in developing nations.

Nothing is simple when dealing with as crafty an adversary as HIV. Scientists are continually searching for its Achilles' heel, and they think they may have found something in a class of compounds known as *entry inhibitors*. As the name suggests, these drugs attempt to thwart infection by preventing the virus from getting into our cells. The strategy is to confuse HIV by releasing "decoys" into the blood. One such decoy is the CD4 molecule, which, when on the surface of a T cell, acts as a docking site for the virus. It is reasoned that HIV will attach to these free CD4s instead of the CD4s on T cells, and infection will be averted.

One type of entry inhibitor furthest along in development is called T-20, a compound that mimics not the CD4 site of the T cell, but rather the gp 41 portion of the HIV protein envelope. It is gp 41 that facilitates fusion of HIV with the cell membrane, allowing admittance into the cell. What T-20 molecules do is bind with uninfected immune cells, thereby denying HIV the opportunity to infect.

Regardless of how they work, what all entry inhibitors share is an ability to thwart the virus outside the cell, before infection occurs. And that, some experts believe, may give them a better chance of dispatching HIV than the currently available antivirals, all of which work inside cells already infected. "Working outside the cell gives them, in theory, a major advantage," says David Ho, the 1996 *Time* Man of the Year, "because cell membranes can present barriers to some drugs, and some have molecules that pump out drugs that manage to get inside." These drugs are also effective in lower doses and safer for patients than the traditional drug cocktail therapies.

Buoyed by the success of these trials, researchers are busy investigating other compounds that would interrupt HIV's reproductive cycle at critical points. One particularly attractive drug would block HIV from inserting its DNA into the host's genome. And then there are the *antisense* drugs that target the actual genetic material, the RNA, of the virus. It works something like this:

The RNA of HIV is single stranded, unlike DNA, which has a complementary strand bonded to it (the famous double helix). One of the primary missions of this single strand of viral RNA is to churn out millions of molecules of a specific protein it was designed to manufacture. But what if biochemists synthesize a tiny stretch of RNA, called *antisense RNA*, that is complementary to a tiny stretch of HIV RNA? Such antisense snippets, when mixed with the virus, will hopefully stick to its RNA and effectively halt viral protein synthesis.

All of the sundry approaches to defeating HIV through pharmaceuticals underscore one central fact: the more we learn of HIV and how it operates the better and more varied our weapons against it can be. Not all drugs that show great promise in the test tube will pan out in clinical trials, for our knowledge of the interaction between HIV and our immune system is incomplete. Yet we have made great strides in slowing down viral replication, adding many years to the lives of those with full-blown AIDS. And until an effective vaccine is developed, antiretroviral drugs will remain the cornerstone of the anti-HIV effort.

Where Did HIV Come From?

The year 1981 will be remembered as a year of infamy, the year the AIDS pandemic struck—not only in America but in Europe and Africa as well. Actually the first AIDS case has been traced to an English sailor who died of the disease way back in 1959. His opportunistic infections so astounded doctors treating him that they froze and saved his blood and tissue samples. Sure enough, when tested decades later, they proved to be HIV-positive.

Before 1959 human blood—that available for testing—seems to have been free of HIV. So where did it come from, and why did it suddenly strike with such a vengeance?

Right from the beginning there has been no shortage of theories concerning the origin of AIDS. Many wild speculations abound. First there were conspiracy theories—either the Soviets or the Americans had genetically engineered a hybrid virus from a human and a sheep retrovirus. The fact that the nucleic acid of HIV was radically different from that of either virus it allegedly derived from did not seem to matter. Nor did the fact that in 1959 the technology for splicing new viruses together simply was not there. And why, pray tell, would any government purposely design a biological warfare germ that had an asymptomatic incubation period averaging nine years?

Another theory that seems to make more sense is that culturing of the poliovirus in the 1950s for the development of a vaccine introduced HIV into the human population. The reasoning goes like this: poliovirus is grown in live monkey cells—live monkey kidney cells, to be precise. Back then it seemed to be the only place they grew well. (Today poliovirus is grown in both monkey and human cells.) Unfortunately, monkeys sometimes harbor SIV, which is remarkably similar to HIV. Couldn't contamination of a polio vaccine with SIV have occurred?

Certainly it could have happened, although that's unlikely. To begin with, SIV is restricted to African monkeys, whereas the monkeys used in the manufacture of polio vaccine came almost exclusively from Asia. And there are other pieces of the puzzle that don't quite fit, such as the time frame and the strain of SIV being implicated. Yet the theory is hard to dismiss outright, and it has gained wide popularity. In fact, several years ago a father of a girl who inexplicably contracted AIDS sued the provider of her polio vaccine.

Although laboratory-grown monkey cells are not the likely source of HIV, it most likely was an SIV from which the AIDS virus evolved. The evolutionary trail, however, is not an easy one to trace. For starters, there are two types of HIV. HIV-1 is the original AIDS virus. It is responsible for the pandemic the world is now experiencing. But in 1985 a second HIV was found and dubbed *HIV-2*. We now know that it is much less virulent than HIV-1, often causing no illness, and is found almost exclusively in Africa. Also, because it seems to be more benign, HIV-2 is probably an older virus that has existed in the human population for centuries. To complicate matters further, there are many different types of SIV, infecting a wide range of primates. African green monkeys, macaques, sooty mangabeys, cynomolgus monkeys, and chimpanzees all have their SIVs. Which if any are related to HIV-1 and HIV-2?

Interestingly, HIV-1 and HIV-2 are related only distantly, sharing a mere 43 percent of their DNA sequences. Compare that with the 75 percent homology between HIV-2 and SIV of the African green monkey. And HIV-2 is so closely related to the SIV of macaques that some scientists took to using a single designation for the two—HIV/SIVmac. What does all this mean? Zoonosis, or the cross-species transmission of virus from primates to humans, has most likely occurred and is probably still occurring. There is also little doubt that such genetic similarity indicates a common ancestry between HIV-2 and the SIVs.

But what about HIV-1—the AIDS virus—and its origins? The evolutionary trail becomes even more tortuous and difficult to follow. When a computer was enlisted to analyze all of the accumulated data, what emerged were six distinct groups or subtypes of HIV-1. Each group, labeled A through F, had its own unique geographic distribution, mode of transmission, and type of infectivity. Subtype B, for example, was the only one found in North America. It was spread easily through homosexual sex and often resulted in opportunistic infections such as PCP and Kaposi's sarcoma. Subtype A, on the other hand, was the AIDS virus of central Africa and India. It was more readily transmitted through heterosexual sex than subtype B and was much more apt to cause chronic diarrhea and a wasting of the body.

Some researchers believe that HIV-1 has existed at a low level in human populations for hundreds of years, and human activity, not biological change, brought on its emergence. But the latest modeling, using the world's fastest supercomputer, Nirvana, at Los Alamos National Laboratory, suggests otherwise. Based on the genetic dissimilarity of the various subtypes and known mutation rates of HIV-1, this virus most likely made the transition from chimpanzees circa 1930. It was then that the chimp SIV crossed over to a new genus and species, perhaps infecting humans when they killed and ate the animals. Whatever its evolutionary past, the present and future of HIV are what most concern virologists.

What Lies Ahead?

AIDS is a most insidious disease. It seeks out and destroys the very cells designed to protect and defend us. Trying to assess our progress in dealing with HIV is like trying to decide if the glass is half full or half empty. To most it would appear half empty. There is no cure for the disease. There is no prophylactic vaccine. To quote Mark Caldwell in his 1993 *Discover* article, "The truth is that nobody really understands what's going on between these invading retroviruses and the host's immune system." As we approach the year 2003, much of what Caldwell said still rings true. Scientists, as yet, don't have a clue as to how HIV kills all the T4 cells it does. A majority of these cells do not even have HIV replicating within them. Several theories have been promulgated. One is that cells, even uninfected ones, can have certain of their genes turned on, causing them, in effect, to commit suicide. The phenomenon, known as *apoptosis*, has its share of proponents. Another belief is that antibodies to viral glycoproteins attack and destroy healthy cells—the old autoimmune theme. In yet a third theory, scientists speculate that perhaps HIV kills the immature cells of the immune system that go on to produce T cells.

Perhaps, perhaps. Meanwhile people keep dying. But there is light at the end of the tunnel. The nations of the world seem finally to be of one mind in their resolve to defeat this scourge on humanity. In 2001 the United

Nations General Assembly convened a session on HIV/AIDS, the first ever devoted to a public health crisis. A global action plan was drafted, one that will require seven to ten billion dollars a year to implement, coming mostly from developed nations. Private individuals and corporations are contributing their resources to fund groups such as the International AIDS Vaccine Initiative (IAVI), a New York–based agency presently financing five companies involved in vaccine research. Its goal is to have eight to twelve vaccines in development by 2007. Bill and Melinda Gates, of Microsoft fame, have created a foundation that has already pumped more than twenty-four billion dollars into promoting health care in the developing world. Much of the investment is aimed at defeating HIV. With AIDS champion Dr. Anthony Fauci at its helm, the National Institute for Allergy and Infectious Diseases (NIAID) created the HIV Vaccine Trials Network (HVTN), with twelve trial sites within the United States and thirteen outside the country. It is working hand-in-glove with Merck and Co. and other vaccine manufacturers.

Hope springs eternal. On the optimistic side, we appear to be on the threshold of discovering new drugs and drug combinations that will greatly slow down, if not halt, the virus in its tracks. We know its genes, and we know its proteins. We know a lot about how they go about their business. It is a multistep affair, and we are attempting to foil the virus at each and every step. Too many great minds and great technologies are at work worldwide for us not to succeed. Let's hope it will not take another two decades.

11

Bioterrorism

Terrorism and deception are weapons not of the strong but of the weak.

—Mohandas K. Gandhi

Terror is the most effective political instrument. I shall not permit myself to be robbed of it simply because a lot of stupid, bourgeois mollycoddles choose to be offended by it.

—Adolf Hitler

Bioterrorism. A bioterror event. These are recently coined terms to denote the use of biological weapons—infectious agents such as bacteria or viruses—to intentionally inflict harm upon others. The definition is usually expanded to include development of biologically derived toxins such as the poisons produced by the bacteria of botulism, tetanus, or gangrene. The concept, however, is not new. Germ warfare is probably as old as disease itself. More than two thousand years ago Scythian archers dipped arrowheads in manure and the flesh of rotting corpses to make their weapons more lethal. In the Middle Ages an army of Tartars employed catapults to hurl corpses infected with the Black Death (plague) over the walls of the besieged city of Kaffa. More recent are the dastardly deeds of Lord Jeffrey Amherst, a respected general of the British forces in North America during the French and Indian War (1754–63). In doing battle with Pontiac, the Ottawa chief, he knowingly and deliberately had his men distribute smallpox-infected blankets and handkerchiefs to the Indians. It subsequently started a deadly epidemic among the highly susceptible population of Native Americans. For his efforts Lord Jeffrey, military hero, became the eponymous founder of a major city in Massachusetts. A university in that same state also bears his name.

By the mid-1900s, science and medicine greatly expanded our knowledge of the deadly microbes with which we share the planet. Sadly, human nature and testosterone being what they are, this wisdom did little to deter our use of pathogens as weapons of mass death. On the contrary. Modern technology merely replaced catapults and blankets to more effectively process and deliver the pathogenic payload.

The Nations

With the advent of modern technology, including a global electronic information "highway" called the World Wide Web, and the proliferation of terrorist groups into an expanding terrorist network—both twentieth-century phenomena—nations began developing germ warfare programs. For both offensive and defensive purposes they created and weaponized deadly microbes and their toxins. The United States, sadly, became one of the key players in this dangerous game.

America: Home of the Brave

In 1942 Franklin D. Roosevelt appointed George W. Merck, president of the giant Merck drug company, to head America's secret germ warfare effort. A company trusted by generations of physicians for supplying them with the knowledge and medications to heal was now involved in a very different enterprise.

Headquarters for research and development of bioweapons (BW) was established at Fort Detrick, a sprawling army base in rural Maryland. It was to remain America's primary germ warfare facility until 1969. In that year, with demonstrations against the Vietnam War on the rise and anti-bioweapons sentiment increasing, President Nixon shut down America's germ warfare program. Only research of a defensive nature would be allowed, and Detrick became the United States Army Medical Research Institute of Infectious Diseases (USAMRIID).

In the early years of Detrick's operation, America's hunt for biological weapons focused on bacterial assassins. It was here that scientists, in the early 1950s, learned to increase the virulence of *Bacillus anthracis*, a bacterium that, if inhaled, causes a usually fatal form of the disease anthrax. One gallon of the new and improved bacillus held up to eight billion lethal doses, enough to kill every man, woman, and child inhabiting the planet. American scientists also solved the more daunting problems of turning living anthrax bacteria into hardy, dormant spores and then weaponizing them in aerosol dispensers. Even General Mills, maker of Cheerios and Wheaties, joined the germ-war effort, constructing a device to spray pathogenic microorganisms continuously from an airplane.

At Fort Detrick, America's hunt for biological weapons focused on other deadly bacteria as well. The causative agents of plague and tularemia were studied. Plague—the Black Death—is a horrific disease that is responsible for several of the worst human die-offs in recorded history. Tularemia might be considered a less virulent, less contagious cousin of plague, with mortality figures in the 35 percent range. At the peak of its operation, the United States was producing 1.6 metric tons of tularemia germs a year.

By the mid-1950s the Pentagon decided to expand operations and start looking seriously at viruses as possible germ weapons. They were, after all, impervious to antibiotics, and some of the most deadly diseases were viral in nature. With these thoughts in mind, Pine Bluff Arsenal was carved out of the woods in Arkansas and set up as a second major lethal germ factory. Its principle function would be to study and ultimately mass-produce viruses for biological warfare.

Working in concert with Detrick, Pine Bluff made a broader selection of bioweapons available. Then in 1958 Castro seized power in Cuba. A communist threat was now only miles off our southeastern coast. The situation worsened in 1962, with the Cuban missile crisis bringing America and Russia to the brink of nuclear war. What to do? A plan was drawn up to invade Cuba and depose Castro. But before any military action, the United States would weaken enemy resistance with a biostrike. One lethal option that was considered involved spraying Cuban troops with botulinum toxin. Synthesized by the bacterium *Clostridium botulinum*, this toxin is the most powerful poison known—ten thousand times more lethal than nerve gas. A glassful of pure toxin could, theoretically, wipe out all human life on the planet. Perhaps this was a bit of overkill, since America merely wanted to incapacitate the Cuban troops before a military attack. So an alternate plan was drawn up, using an aerosolized cocktail of two germs and one toxin. They would work sequentially, producing illness and debilitation within several hours of the spraying, and lasting up to three weeks.

The toxin of the mixture was staphylococcal enterotoxin B (SEB), secreted by a staph bacterium and a main cause of common food poisoning. Its symptoms—chills, headache, muscle pain, coughing, and high fever—would begin three to twelve hours after inhaling the poisonous vapors. The two germs employed were a virus that causes a form of encephalitis and a rickettsia (tiny bacterium approaching the size of a viral particle) that is the agent of Q fever. Encephalitis would present as nausea and diarrhea, with a spiking fever of up to 105°F, followed by weeks of weakness and malaise. Q fever, after a ten- to twenty-day incubation period, produces two weeks of debilitating headaches, chills, hallucinations, facial pain, and fever. In short, the blend of bugs and poison should not kill its victims but just make them feel like dying. It was predicted that many of Cuba's population of seven million would fall ill, about 1 percent—or seventy thousand—fatally so. The beauty of the attack lay in the fact that it was not contagious and the microbial spray would dissipate before American soldiers arrived, leaving in its wake a helpless Cuban military.

Both the virus and rickettsia were grown in fertilized chick eggs (since both required living cells for growth), almost half a million of them, producing hundreds of gallons of pathogenic agent. But ultimately, saner heads prevailed, and the mission was scrapped.

Eisenhower considered incapacitating biological agents a "splendid idea," and funding for bioweapons research and development increased significantly under his presidency and that of John F. Kennedy. Then, in 1969, President Nixon abruptly pulled the plug on our offensive bioweapons program. But the CIA, even after Nixon's ban, kept a small arsenal of germs and toxins, capable of sickening and/or killing millions of people. This included one hundred grams of smallpox virus, a nightmare pathogen that the United States had researched as a weapon of mass annihilation, even as it led the effort to wipe out the terrible scourge worldwide.

Several years later, 139 nations would follow America's lead and join the United States in banning bioweapons when, in 1972, they signed and ratified the Biological and Toxin Weapons Convention. The agreement called for termination of all offensive weapons research and development, as well as destruction of all existing stockpiles of agents by 1975. Sadly, the treaty was unenforceable and many nations did not fully comply, including America. Ronald Reagan, fearing that Soviets were bioengineering new superbugs (and they were), by splicing genes from one bacterium or virus to another, interpreted the 1972 accord quite liberally. He considered almost any research, no matter how ominous, to be of a defensive nature. In the service of protecting American citizenry and armed servicemen, Pentagon research included 51 projects aimed at making novel pathogens, 32 at boosting toxin production, 23 at defeating vaccines, 14 at inhibiting diagnosis, and 3 at outwitting protective drugs. Nothing like a treaty banning bioweapons to keep the world safe!

In one experiment, an American scientist at Stanford University moved a dangerous gene from a virulent bacterium related to plague into the harmless gut bacterium *Escherichia coli*, creating a superbug that attacked human cells. This was, of course, research of a purely defensive nature.

Splicing of genes from one microbe to another to create novel life forms was a technology that dated back to the mid-1970s. In 1978 the gene producing human insulin had been inserted into ubiquitous *E. coli*. The bacteria were then grown in huge vats and the insulin they manufactured was harvested. No longer did diabetics have to rely on live sheep and pigs for their lifesaving hormone. Unfortunately, the potential for genetic engineering as a tool of bioterrorism was almost limitless. This terrified President Clinton, who particularly feared the ability of rogue nations such as Iraq to manipulate genes. The United States must concentrate its efforts on defense against such a biological threat. Toward this end he poured hundreds of millions of dollars for biodefense into the Defense Advanced Research Projects Agency (DARPA). The money was used to fund projects aimed at finding new antibacterial and antiviral agents, as well as new and improved vaccines. One study focused on the search for gene vaccines—particular genes of a pathogen that can be injected into people. The genes would incorporate into body cells and start the production of proteins specific to that germ—proteins that would sensitize the immune system against said pathogen.

Without question, America was a serious bioweaponeer through the middle decades of the twentieth century. By 1970, however, the United States had significantly reduced efforts to weaponize germs and their toxins. Much of the work that continued of an offensive nature was fueled by the large-scale germ war operations of Russia, operations that continued unimpeded by any treaties the nation had signed.

Russia: Moscow's Microbes

The endeavors of America to transform pathogenic microorganisms into armaments paled in comparison to that of the U.S.S.R. The Soviet program of weaponizing germs was the earliest of any nation, beginning in the 1920s and '30s and growing rapidly under the dictatorship of Stalin. But it was after World War II that Moscow really became serious about producing germs for war. Through the 1940s and '50s many sites were set up throughout the countryside to develop biological weapons—Sverdlovsk and Stepnogorsk specialized in anthrax, others in smallpox or plague. Collectively, all the germ warfare facilities came to be called the *Biopreparat*—a biological war machine that, at its peak in the 1980s, employed sixty thousand people in more than one hundred locations. It was by far the most massive bioweapons construct any country ever created.

One favorite microbe of the Russians, as with the Americans, was *B. anthracis*. It was while experimenting with this deadly bacterium in Sverdlovsk that seventy-nine people reportedly became mysteriously ill in the nearby countryside, sixty-eight of them dying. The cause—anthrax. Moscow blamed it on tainted meat, but after the fall of communism in 1991, Boris Yeltsin admitted it was a military research accident. *B. anthracis* spores had escaped into the air one spring day in 1979 and gotten people sick as far as fifty miles from the source of the mishap.

Before the Soviet shutdown of Biopreparat—twenty years after it had signed the Biological Weapons Convention of 1972—the Russians developed more than two thousand strains of anthrax alone. Different strains, if dissimilar enough, often require different vaccines to confer immunity, much as the flu virus of this year requires a different vaccine than the one of a year ago. Of the two thousand strains, a number were and still are of particular concern, either for having had their virulence increased several-fold, or for exhibiting antibiotic resistance. According to Ken Alibek, the top man in the Biopreparat for twenty years, and a defector to the United States in 1992, Moscow maintained forty-five hundred metric tons of anthrax at all times. Several pounds of purified *B. anthracis* could wipe out a small city. It was grown in huge twenty-ton fermentation vats that rose four stories high. What in blazes were they going to do with forty-five hundred metric tons—kill every American one hundred times?

By 1980 the Soviets had embarked on a strategy with two distinct objectives. One was the production of old-fashioned germs, affectionately referred to by scientists as oldie-moldies. Plague bacteria (*Y. pestis*) was such an oldie-moldie, and huge quantities—on the order of fifteen hundred metric tons—was manufactured and stockpiled. The second focus of the U.S.S.R.'s germ war effort was futuristic research into bioengineered pathogens. Unlike Western nations, which, to some degree, abided by the dictums of the 1972 Biological Weapons Convention, Moscow chose to completely flaunt its directives. This proved most unfortunate for the United States and its allies, since the 1970s and '80s were a time of significant discoveries in the biology of the cell. Genes and the DNA of which they are constructed were being studied and manipulated in the laboratory in fantastic ways, creating cellular chimera—hybrids with genes from two or more organisms. It was not long before this new biotechnology found its way to the Biopreparat of Russia. Germs could now be made hardier, more lethal, more resistant to treatment, and immune to vaccine. In 1984, sources claimed that Moscow had put the genes from cobra snake cells into otherwise harmless viruses and bacteria, giving them the ability to produce deadly venom in a victim's body.

Russia also succeeded, where America had failed, in creating a new, genetically improved version of the Black Death, impervious to existing vaccines and antibiotics. Then the Soviets packed a dry, powdered form of this superplague into bombs, warheads of intercontinental ballistic missiles (ICBMs), and artillery shells. The gloves were coming off. Perhaps Ronald Reagan's "Evil Empire" was precisely that.

Beginning in 1980, Soviet scientists undertook an aggressive campaign to produce hundreds of tons of smallpox virus and then adapt the virus for deployment in bombs and ICBMs. Smallpox is acknowledged by germ warfare experts to be the most dangerous and potentially devastating of all bioweapons, and mass-producing such huge quantities is beyond human comprehension. In contrast, the United States had done virtually nothing to weaponize this nightmare germ.

Much of the work on smallpox was done at Vector (now the State Research Center of Virology and Biotechnology), Moscow's giant institute in remote Siberia that specialized in weaponizing the world's deadliest viruses. The facility housed 120 different smallpox isolates and another 10,000 specimens of the world's most lethal and exotic viral agents. Vector had sent an expedition to Siberian villages to dig up long-frozen bodies of smallpox victims from the turn of the century, in hopes of retrieving viable samples of the virus. Moscow also sent scientists to Africa to collect the viruses of Ebola and Marburg—diseases with extremely high mortality that literally liquefy the internal organs, causing horrendous bleed-outs (see Chapter 7, "Emerging Viruses"). The expectation was that Vector researchers could develop a smallpox/Marburg hybrid. Marburg was not very contagious, but was extremely deadly, and no vaccine or cure existed. Smallpox was more infectious, but there was a vaccine. First there would be smallpox symptoms, and then Marburg would hit. Craig Venter, the American biogeneticist who was instrumental in mapping the human genome, said such a melding of monster viruses was very possible. The world's worst-ever disease could be made even more frightful.

In 1988 a Soviet scientist died of Marburg. It was discovered, upon isolation of the virus, that it had mutated to a more lethal form. What good fortune for the Soviets, who quickly weaponized it.

Top Russian DNA-recombination scientists who defected in the early 1990s to both the United States and Britain told of other horror stories. In the late 1970s, Sergei Popov and his Vector colleagues inserted genes for myelin proteins and protein fragments into viruses. Myelin sheaths coat and insulate human nerve cells. In the autoimmune disorder multiple sclerosis, our own immune system attacks and destroys this myelin. Russia was attempting to invent an infectious microorganism that triggered such an autoimmune condition. Apparently they succeeded, engineering a bug that destroyed nervous tissue, causing brain damage and death in experimental animals—an induced, rapid-onset MS.

The bacterium that causes Legionnaires' disease was also equipped with myelin protein genes. Infected guinea pigs first contracted Legionnaires', a pneumonia with 20 to 25 percent mortality rate if untreated (see Chapter 5, "New Kids on the Block"), followed by brain damage, paralysis, and death. Mortality rates approached 100 percent. Very infectious as well as virulent, thankfully it was never turned into a weapon.

In 1993, Russia successfully inserted virulence genes from a bacterium called *B. cereus* into their old favorite, the anthrax microbe. *B. cereus* can be serious, attacking red blood cells, although it is normally not fatal. When combined with *B. anthracis*, however, it proved eminently so, killing all the hamsters that were infected, even those given the Russian anthrax vaccine. These superbugs, as well as Marburg, Ebola, and others, were tested on lab animals in fifty-foot-high aerosol chambers. Moscow even open-air tested anthrax, tularemia, Q fever, brucellosis, glanders, plague, and possibly smallpox on a remote island in the Aral Sea called Renaissance Island. It was here that the Soviets buried tons of anthrax spores in steel canisters after "decontaminating" them with bleach. It is doubtful that all the anthrax was rendered harmless. I would not be vacationing on Renaissance Island anytime soon.

Although Russia never did and probably never will completely discontinue its search for ever-more-lethal pathogens, Yeltsin did begin dismantling the Soviet biological warfare machine after the fall of Gorbachev and his party. But with the collapse of the communist government, other concerns surfaced. Hundreds of Russian scientists were now unemployed; scientists with access to deadly germs and the know-how to weaponize them. Some would defect to the West and find gainful employment there. Many, however, would sell their lethal contraband and expertise to the highest bidder. In postcommunist, poverty-stricken Russia, security for deadly germs was almost nonexistent. According to Judith Miller, Stephen Engelberg, and William Broad, writers of *Germs*, "a collection of more than 1,000 lethal germ strains was protected only by a rickety wooden door and a single skeleton-key lock." Enough plague to depopulate the entire region sat unsecured in a rusty pea can.

Almost certainly, smallpox from the Vector plant walked during the 1990s. Dr. Peter Jahrling, a distinguished infectious diseases expert at USAMRIID, had this to say after a tour of the site, "The only apparent security was one pimply-faced kid who looked about fourteen with a Kaleshnikov rifle" (*Living Terrors*, by Michael T. Osterholm and John Schwartz).

Which countries were we most concerned about as benefactors of Russia's crumbling economy? Iraq was at the top of a short list of rogue nations that included Iran, North Korea, and South Africa along with well-financed terrorist groups such as the al Qaeda network of Muslim fanatic Osama bin Laden.

Iraq: Saddam Country

Precisely when Iraq began to seriously consider germs as potential weapons is hard to say. It was certainly well after both the U.S.S.R. and America, and their bioweapons program did not really get rolling until the early 1980s. But once started, it rapidly became the most advanced and most extensive in the Arab world. A drain of technological expertise from the former U.S.S.R surely aided their cause. It is also believed that Iraq's sudden rise to prominence was due, in large measure, to training many Iraqis received at Western universities and medical facilities. Iraq's top bioweapons expert, Rihab Taha—also known as Dr. Germ—is a forty-eight-year-old biochemist who was educated in England.

America even supplied Saddam Hussein, Iraqi president, with the bugs. In 1986 the American Type Culture Collection (ATCC) sold an assortment of pathogens to the University of Baghdad. They included three anthrax strains, five types of botulinum, and three variants of brucella, the causative agent of a serious but not normally fatal disease called brucellosis. The ATCC, a scientific supply company in the suburbs of Washington, D.C., was and still is the world's largest germ repository. Their inventory included the most lethal variants of every conceivable pathogen (excluding smallpox).

Two years later, in 1988, the ATCC once again filled and delivered an order from Iraq. This time eleven different germ strains were sent, four of which were anthrax. At the time there seemed little reason to deny Iraq, which America viewed as an ally in its hostilities with Iran. But by early 1989 a ban was placed on sale of anthrax and dozens of other pathogens to Iraq as well as Iran, Libya, and Syria, all of which were suspected of developing germ weapons. Restrictions on the sale of pathogens was further tightened when, in 1995, American white supremacist Larry Wayne

Harris ordered and received three vials of freeze-dried bubonic plague bacteria from the ATCC. Luckily, they turned out to be innocuous vaccine strains.

With the ATCC no longer available to rogue nations and terrorist groups as supplier of deadly germs, Iraq had to turn to new sources. Not a problem. The World Directory of Collections of Cultures and Microorganisms lists some 450 such repositories worldwide, and according to Pulitzer Prize–winning writer Laurie Garrett, "more than fifty of them sold anthrax, sixty-four would sell the organism that causes typhoid fever, and thirty-four offered the bacterium that produces botulinum toxin. These businesses—many of which take orders over the Internet—can be found in more than sixty nations including China, Bulgaria, Turkey, Argentina, and Iran. Eighteen repositories, located in fifteen different countries traded in plague bacteria" (*Living Terrors*, Osterholm and Schwartz). It is also interesting to note that a recent survey by the American Society of Microbiology found 22 percent of nearly fifteen hundred academic institutions work with pathogenic microorganisms and toxins that could be used in biological weapons development. A determined terrorist could hire on at one of these labs as a student or technician and obtain a starter culture.

By the late 1980s, American intelligence knew that Iraq was constructing a biological arsenal under the guise of legitimate research into biopesticides. Of particular interest to Saddam Hussein were the two oldie-moldies, anthrax and botulism. Through the 1980s Baghdad also dabbled in molecular biology, doing research into the genetic engineering of pathogens. A 1990 report from *Armed Forces Medical Intelligence* summed up the Iraq threat as "a mature offensive BW program."

At the height of Iraq's germ weaponization, in 1991, Baghdad had eight industrial-sized facilities, producing eighty-five thousand liters of anthrax germs, three hundred thousand liters of botulinum toxin, and twenty-two hundred liters of cancer-causing aflatoxin, which is derived from a fungus. There were also substantial amounts of *V. cholerae* (cholera), staphylococcus enterotoxin B, and *Cl. perfringens* or its toxin (gas gangrene). Twenty-five SCUD missile warheads were filled with anthrax, botulinum, and aflatoxin. Three hundred bombs had various and sundry biological agents. And a two-thousand-liter aircraft-mounted aerosol spray tank was at the ready.

In 1990 Saddam Hussein purchased forty top-of-the-line aerosol generators capable of dispersing anthrax spores at the incredible rate of eight hundred gallons an hour, either in liquid form or as a dry, powdered agent. Each device was compact enough to fit on a truck, small boat, or single-engine plane. There is also reason to believe that Hussein subsequently established communication with Osama bin Laden and may have offered bioterror knowledge and supplies to his terrorist organization, al Qaeda.

Like other late-twentieth-century bioweaponeer nations, Iraq began experimenting with viruses. One viral agent was camelpox, which is a relative of smallpox. Rotavirus, a common cause of severe diarrhea, and hemorrhagic conjunctivitis, an affliction causing temporary blindness, were also investigated.

After the Persian Gulf War, Iraq was subjected to routine inspections by the United Nations Special Commission—UNSCOM. The mission of this international body, which incorporated military personnel as well as scientists, was to search for and uncover evidence of chemical, biological, and/or nuclear weapons development. What soon became clear was that the war itself had destroyed little, if any, of Hussein's biological armaments. And through all the investigations, which ended in December 1998, when UNSCOM inspectors were forced to pull out of Iraq, it was this weapons arsenal that Hussein most fiercely guarded and protected. He went so far as to bury germ-filled bombs a meter underground before inspection of a facility at Al Hakim. Production lines were only temporarily shut down during such inspections. At one point, in 1995, Baghdad admitted making thousands of gallons of germ weapons. Under UNSCOM supervision, some of its anthrax and botulism cache was destroyed, but only a small fraction, experts believe.

To date, it is feared that the United Nations has been totally unsuccessful in dismantling any of Saddam Hussein's biowarfare capabilities. Following UNSCOM's pullout, Iraq's dictator began aggressively stockpiling materials, converting commercial production facilities for bioterror use. By the late 1990s Iraq sought to upgrade its germ warfare operations by shopping around Russia for bioweapons experts with gene recombination skills. Much information is also available on the Internet. In short, Iraq remains a serious bioterror threat to Israel and the West, as well as other Arab nations—and was accurately described by U.S. President George W. Bush as part of an "axis of evil."

The Germs

Biological weapons are the poor man's nukes. In 1993 the congressional Office of Technology Assessment (OTA) came to the shocking conclusion that "100 kg of anthrax spores (about 220 pounds) would be more lethal than a SCUDlike missile carrying a hydrogen bomb." The airplane, dispersing its deadly germ cargo on a clear night in Washington, D.C., would wipe out 1 to 3 million people as compared to an H-bomb kill of .6 to 1.9 million. The numbers for smallpox would be even more devastating. Pound for pound, as well as dollar for dollar, bioweapons outkill nuclear ones many times over—"$1,500 of nuclear killing power would set an anthrax assailant back one cent" (*Living Terrors*, Osterholm and Schwartz). Small wonder as many as twenty-five nations and assorted terrorist groups have found germ warfare attractive enough to begin bioweapons production, and this in spite of the international ban on such endeavors. Syria, Libya, South Africa, North Korea, Iraq, Sudan, Cuba, and China are but a few of the countries amassing germ weapons. And there are hundreds of germs to choose from—germs that can be cultured and fashioned into insidious instruments of death.

A NATO handbook lists thirty-one potential biological agents of war, some more effectively grown and dispersed than others, to affect mass annihilation. The four highest on NATO's list are smallpox, plague, anthrax, and botulism. In 1998, Johns Hopkins Center for Civilian Biodefense Studies listed smallpox and anthrax as those germ weapons with the greatest potential for inflicting massive numbers of casualties.

What makes these germs more serious threats than the others? When assessing a microorganism's weapon potential, several factors come into play. The most important are its killing power, its ease of delivery, and its stability. Let us look at the worst of the worst.

Anthrax

When the Lord visited his deadly plague upon the cattle of Pharaoh, as recounted in Exodus, it was most certainly anthrax. The disease is contracted when grazing animals inhale or ingest anthrax spores found in soil. Humans acquire anthrax naturally when they come into close contact with infected animals, usually through the handling of contaminated wool, animal hides, or animal hair products (such as brushes). In mid–nineteenth-century Europe it went by the names "woolsorter's" or "ragpicker's" disease. Anthrax is an unlikely bioweapon. Throughout history it has not been a prolific killer of humans. The worst-ever documented outbreak of anthrax occurred in 1979, when ten kilograms (twenty-two pounds) of spores escaped into the air from a Russian military institution. Supposedly, sixty-eight out of seventy-nine infected people in the nearby countryside perished. Certainly not a die-off of epidemic proportions, and naturally occurring outbreaks kill far fewer. The common flu routinely kills twenty thousand Americans annually. Why then have so many nations and terrorist groups focused on this microbe, which is not contagious, rarely if ever spreading from person to person?

In a word, *durability*. *B. anthracis* is one of only a handful of seriously pathogenic bacteria that produce spores. Living microbes are fragile things and die or lose virulence quite readily. Heat, cold, dryness, gloom of night easily bring on their demise. But when living conditions become intolerable for *B. anthracis*, it creates a thick, impervious coat around itself and slips into a state of suspended animation called *dormancy*. As a spore, the anthrax bacillus can survive tremendous extremes of temperature, radiation, and aridity for many decades, suddenly springing to life when living conditions improve.

Anthrax can also be a very deadly disease, which is another of its selling points as a bioterror weapon. There are actually three forms of anthrax infection, depending on the bacteria's route of entry into the human body:

Skin or cutaneous anthrax. This is the most common manifestation of the disease, accounting for 95 percent of all anthrax cases. Contraction occurs through a cut or other break in the skin. Initially a small, itchy bump appears, which resembles a spider bite and may be accompanied by a localized rash. The bacillus is now rapidly multiplying and releasing potent toxins that cause a fluid-filled pustule to develop. As toxins continue killing healthy tissue over the next few days, the lesion transforms into a painless ulcer one to three centimeters (.4 to 1.2 inches) in diameter and black in the center. Lymph glands in the adjacent area may swell and become tender as systemic symptoms such as fever and myalgia (muscle pain) present themselves. If left untreated, the mortality rate is about 20 percent. With antibiotic therapy, deaths are rare.

Gastrointestinal anthrax. There is an incubation period of one to seven days, following ingestion of raw or undercooked meat contaminated with anthrax bacteria or bacterial spores. *B. anthracis* matures and replicates within the intestine, releasing deadly toxins that produce lesions and acute inflammation. Patients present with severe abdominal pain, nausea, vomiting (sometimes bloody), and bloody diarrhea, accompanied by fever. The disease can also affect the upper GI tract, creating lesions at the base of the tongue and a bad sore throat with fever. If left untreated, 25 to 60 percent of GI cases result in death. It is, however, a rare form of anthrax.

Inhalation or pulmonary anthrax. This is the deadliest form of the disease, killing 90 percent of those victims who are untreated. Antibiotics can be effective, but must be administered in the first days after infection. The incubation period for inhalation anthrax among humans is unclear. Typically the disease presents within one to seven days, but inhaled spores can remain dormant in the lungs for up to sixty days and possibly longer in rare instances. Initial symptoms resemble those of a common cold or the flu—sore throat, mild fever, muscle aches, malaise, and a nonproductive cough. After several days, as bacterial toxins do their damage, the symptoms progress to high fever and a difficulty in breathing as the lungs fill with fluid. Death soon follows as toxic shock leads to a rapid drop in blood pressure and organ failure.

With anthrax, it is not the bacteria that wreak havoc, but rather the poisons they produce. There are three toxins in all, and they work in concert, first attaching to human cell membranes and then entering the cell. A favorite target of these killer chemicals is the macrophage, a white blood cell of the immune system whose job it is to attack and destroy germs by literally eating them. But *B. anthracis*, after being ingested, is able to survive and even multiply within these cells, much as HIV does. Macrophages then carry their deadly intruders throughout the body, where release of anthrax toxins produce systemic disease and death.

Stability and high mortality are the strengths of *B. anthracis* when considered as a bioweapon. According to a World Health Organization (WHO) report, fifty kilograms (about 110 pounds) of properly prepared anthrax spores, released for two kilometers (1.25 miles) over a city of a half million residents, would cause 125,000 casualties and 95,000 deaths.

Thankfully, however, anthrax also has drawbacks as an agent of bioterror. First, it can be treated successfully with antibiotics. A protective vaccine even exists that can provide immunity. Second, the disease is not spread person-to-person, the significance of which cannot be overstated. Any assault using B. *anthracis* as a germ weapon can and will be contained within the confines of the initial attack parameters. The destruction and loss of human life is self-limiting because there will be no secondary and tertiary waves of infection spreading the disease, each wave more severe and widespread than the last.

In order to confirm anthrax infection, initial clinical assessment must be confirmed through laboratory findings. A definitive test is the culturing of the bacillus from blood, spinal fluid, or skin lesions. Nasal swab cultures do not constitute diagnostic proof of infection. A person with a negative nose culture may have breathed anthrax spores deeply into his or her lungs. Conversely, a positive nose culture does not tell whether a sufficient number of spores have entered the lungs or skin to produce disease.

Direct microscopic examination of suspected fluids or tissues can also reveal the characteristically shaped and stained anthrax bacillus. More sophisticated methods of identification employ fluorescent antibodies, which tag the proper bugs if they are present in any body tissues or secretions. Even DNA fingerprinting has come out of the forensic lab, to be used for rapid identification of anthrax bacteria. This state-of-the-art science uses a technique called *PCR* (*polymerase chain reaction*), which amplifies the genetic material of any microorganisms lurking in a sample of blood. The bacterial DNA can then be analyzed, in much the same way as the DNA of a suspected rapist or murderer is analyzed. Confirmation is possible in as little as thirty minutes.

The treatments currently available to anthrax victims and those potentially exposed to the bacillus are any of a number of antibiotics. The two medications of choice are ciprofloxacin (Cipro) and doxycycline. A prescribed therapy regimen is two tablets a day for a period of ten days in cases of suspected exposure and sixty days for confirmed exposure. Both pharmaceuticals have mild to moderate side effects, those of Cipro being more severe. These commonly include rash, headache, restlessness, and nausea, accompanied by vomiting and diarrhea.

The prophylactic vaccine currently in use has been available since the late 1950s and early '60s. It is manufactured by only one company, Bioport Corp. of Lansing, Michigan, and consists of a substance called *protective antigen*. The antigen, produced by a harmless strain of *B. anthracis*, is filtered from the growth medium and then purified. No whole bacteria, either living or dead, are present in the final product. The vaccine is administered as a series of six inoculations over a period of eighteen months. Annual booster doses are required for ongoing protection. Anthrax Vaccine Adsorbed (AVA), as it is officially known, is not, however, presently available to the general public. Only the military and at-risk veterinarians, lab workers, and livestock handlers qualify for vaccination.

In 2001, following a bioterror release of anthrax spores via envelopes sent through the mail, workers at contaminated postal facilities in the United States were also offered the vaccine. Most declined, fearing adverse reactions to the inoculations. Their fears were well-founded. When 150,000 soldiers were vaccinated during the Persian Gulf War with Iraq, many complained of muscle and joint pain and memory loss. Symptoms similar to chronic fatigue have also been reported, mostly by women. Some feel this constellation of health problems, known as Gulf War Syndrome, is the result of anthrax vaccination. Government officials deny this, citing eighteen separate studies that showed the vaccine to be safe. But the plant that makes the vaccine was shut down by the FDA in 1999 for thirty violations involving safety and sterility problems. It is plausible that materials such as bits of bacterial cell wall could contaminate the vaccine and cause undesirable side effects. Only recently, in early 2002, did Bioport finally receive FDA approval to resume vaccine production. There is also the very real possibility that the vaccine would be ineffective against strains of anthrax (and there are many) that bioterror groups might employ.

All things considered, anthrax is a darn good bioweapon. It pales, however, in comparison to smallpox.

Smallpox

In A.D. 165 a horrific smallpox epidemic swept through the Roman Empire. At its height, two thousand people a day were dying in Rome alone. It raged for fifteen years, killing one-third of Italy's population. Four to seven million Europeans perished before the pandemic subsided. Ever since that time, smallpox has waxed and waned throughout the world, wiping out a half billion people in the twentieth century until its eradication in 1977. No other germ (save perhaps the bacillus of tuberculosis) has killed more people. Those lost in all the world's wars are but a fraction of the victims felled by variola—the smallpox virus.

As a possible bioweapon, smallpox has no peer. It is the nightmare to end all nightmares. Say "worst case scenario" to any biodefense expert and you will get a one-word reply: smallpox. The nineteenth-century historian Thomas Babington Macaulay called it "the most terrible of the ministers of death."

What is it about this rather large (for a virus), brick-shaped particle that makes it such a terrifying and prolific exterminator of human life? The most dire feature of smallpox is the ease with which it spreads from person to person. Although not as explosively contagious as the measles or the flu, inhalation of even a few viral particles can result in disease. And an infected person exhales thousands of viruses with each breath.

The disease typically has a long incubation period—ten to fourteen days. During that time, the victim feels fine, but the virus is slowly and inexorably multiplying. Early symptoms include high fever, fatigue, and head- and backaches. These are standard flu symptoms as well, so why suspect a disease that has not existed for twenty-five years and that no doctor has ever seen? When hearing hoofbeats in Central Park, don't look for zebras.

Two to three days later, a red rash appears, first on the mouth, throat, and face, then on the arms and legs, appearing last on the torso. Lesions are also less numerous on the torso. This distribution and sequence of emergence is important, since it distinguishes smallpox from chicken pox, which is more severe on the torso. The rash soon develops into bulletlike, tense, pus-filled blisters that are raised and yet deeply imbedded in the skin. It gives the skin a cobblestone appearance. If one is lucky, by the second week of the rash the pustules begin to crust and dry out. Scabs eventually form, which fall off in three to four weeks. The victim has survived, a bit facially pockmarked but alive to tell the tale.

In severe smallpox, the lesions become so numerous that they fuse into a sheetlike layer across the body. The skin then separates from the underlying tissue, an incredibly painful event called "splitting" of the skin, in which the victim feels as if on fire. These patients almost invariably die.

Yet another outcome of variola infection—called the *black pox*—results in skin lesions turning black as hemorrhaging occurs. The skin can actually slip off the body in sheets. Black, unclotted blood runs from every orifice as the virus disintegrates the linings of the throat, stomach, intestines, rectum, and vagina. It is 100 percent fatal.

About one-third of all people contracting smallpox will die. It is this high level of mortality, coupled with a long incubation period and ease of transmission that conspire to make the variola virus an ideal bioweapon. Communist Russia produced twenty tons of smallpox, to be weaponized in missile warheads. Manufacture of such vast quantities was redundant and utterly foolish. Today's bioterrorist will sneak into a crowded mall or airport terminal with an aerosol device no larger than a pack of cigarettes and loaded with several tablespoons of infectious liquid. Operating on a small battery, it will spray an invisible mist of one- to five-micron-size particles into the atmosphere. Soon the entire building is filled with microscopic, virus-laden droplets drifting aimlessly until inhaled deeply into the lungs.

Initially one thousand smallpox cases might result, but let us be conservative in our estimate and begin with one hundred. This represents the first wave of contagion. Roughly two weeks after exposure, symptoms appear. Meanwhile, each infected person has had opportunity to transmit the disease to many others, some in places far from ground zero. How rapidly the disease will mushroom is a matter of conjecture. It was once believed that each primary case could result in hundreds of secondary cases. The CDC now feels this to be greatly overstated, since smallpox victims, by the time they become rabidly contagious, are usually far too ill to be out and about infecting others. Each initial victim probably creates only several new cases. But no one really knows, and the amplification factor could easily be ten. A first wave of one hundred smallpox cases would be followed by an incubation period lull and then a second wave of smallpox that has increased exponentially to more than one thousand. The third wave would explode two weeks later, with more than ten thousand falling victim and no end in sight.

The preceding scenario points out the need for rapid diagnosis of the disease. Doctors might first suspect the flu, or chicken pox, or an allergic reaction, and tests for these illnesses would be performed. When they turned up negative, and smallpox was strongly suspected, samples would have to be sent to either the CDC in Atlanta, Georgia, or USAMRIID in Maryland. These two labs are the only places in the United States equipped to identify variola virus in body tissues or fluids. Hopefully hospitals would isolate the early cases presumptively until smallpox was confirmed. Once confirmed, mandatory quarantine and a massive "ring" vaccination program would kick in. A circle would be drawn on a map, with the initial cases at its center. All people within the circle would be inoculated in an effort to stop transmission dead in its tracks.

Let me reiterate—smallpox is serious stuff. Unlike bacterial diseases, viral infections such as smallpox are untreatable with antibiotics. Some antiviral drugs such as Cidofovir, discovered in the decades-long battle against AIDS, have demonstrated a degree of success against smallpox, and hopefully within a few years others will become available that can ameliorate smallpox symptoms and improve chances of survival. But only the CDC in Atlanta has access to the smallpox virus, which makes research and development by other labs virtually impossible.

Even the smallpox vaccine is problematic. It has been around for two hundred years and is highly effective in conferring immunity to the disease. Regrettably, however, no one knows how long that immunity lasts. Ten years is the accepted number, and therein lies the dilemma. The United States, along with many other nations, stopped inoculating in the early 1970s, when smallpox was no longer considered a natural disease threat. For thirty years, no American has been vaccinated. When it comes to smallpox, we are all like the early Native Americans, naive and susceptible.

To make matters worse, as the year 2002 began, America had only fifteen million doses of vaccine. It had been made by the pharmaceutical giant Wyeth-Ayerst twenty-five to thirty years ago by a traditional method. Calves had their bellies scratched with the cowpox virus, vaccinia (a close relative of smallpox), causing pustules to develop. The calves were then killed, hung up on hooks and the blood drained from them. Pus was scraped from their sores and freeze-dried. The vaccine is calf pus, containing live vaccinia virus and looking, for all the world, like nose snot.

About half of this decades-old vaccine supply had been invaded by moisture and was probably worthless. That left 7.5 million doses. According to Donald A. Henderson, the man who directed WHO's eradication of smallpox and the globe's foremost authority on the disease, "a hundred million doses of vaccine would be needed in the United States alone to stop a surging outbreak triggered by a hundred initial cases from a bioterror event."

Seven and a half million doses of vaccine fell woefully short of the number needed to protect American citizens. On September 20, 2000, the CDC had entered into an agreement with OraVax to produce a new smallpox vaccine. Like the older version used to eradicate smallpox, it would contain live cowpox virus, but modern vaccine preparation techniques would be employed, guaranteeing a safer product. Unfortunately, delivery of the first full-scale production lots was not expected until 2004. This was unacceptable in light of recent bioterror happenings. More vaccine was needed in a hurry, prompting President George W. Bush's administration to contract for an immediate additional 209 million doses, to be manufactured and stockpiled by the end of 2002. It was also believed that the old vaccine could be stretched through dilution and still be effective, yielding an additional sixty million doses, and bringing the total close to three hundred million—roughly one dose for every American.

Once the U.S. government has all the vaccine it believes it needs, the question is what to do with it. Some experts favor routine vaccination for everyone preemptively. Others would reserve the vaccine to use only in the event of an outbreak. To begin with, the vaccine is not completely safe— few vaccines are. In the United States, in 1968, some fourteen million people received the vaccine. There were 572 adverse reactions, resulting in nine deaths. That's nearly twice the number of fatalities from the fall 2001 anthrax attack. The vaccine is also effective in conferring immunity to the disease, or lessening its severity, if given as late as four days after exposure to the virus. Beyond the four-day window to protect, a measure of prophylaxis is still available if vaccination is coupled with the administering of vaccinia immune globulin. So why rush to vaccinate against an agent that in all probability will never be used?

Weighing all the pros and cons of mass vaccination, in June 2002 a federal health advisory panel recommended smallpox vaccination only for specially created federal, state, and local bioterrorism response teams. Each team, of which there would be about 280 nationally, would consist of diagnostic lab scientists, disease investigators, doctors, nurses, and law enforcement personnel.

It is truly tragic that a disease the world spent fifteen years and hundreds of millions of dollars (billions by today's costs) to eradicate may well return as a bioterrorist's weapon. What may save us from a smallpox attack is the difficulty an individual terrorist might encounter in attempting to acquire the variola virus. Although a dozen or more rogue nations and large terrorist networks may have the bug, it is not an easy microbe to come by. Officially, it exists in only two repositories: the CDC in Atlanta, Georgia, and Vector in Siberia. This, however, is not true of the Black Death, a disease that still occurs naturally throughout much of the world, including the United States.

Plague

Plague, in its broadest sense, refers to any horrific and widespread contagion. But to a person of medicine, it can mean only one thing, the Black Death. It is a disease with quite a history. During the first three centuries A.D. and culminating in the Plague of Justinian (A.D. 540–590) it ravaged the Roman Empire, and in so doing, allowed Christianity, with its healing through divine intervention and its promise of life eternal to establish itself as a world force. The infamous Black Death of Europe (1346–61) killed twenty-four million—nearly one-third of that continent's population—and hastened the demise of feudalism and the Middle Ages. Many Jews were persecuted and exterminated as purveyors of the pestilence. In 1665–66 it returned yet a third time as the Great Plague of London. At its peak, each week the Black Death was killing more than seven thousand citizens of the city on the Thames.

The disease is caused by a rod-shaped bacterium, a bacillus, called *Yersinia pestis*, which resides naturally in rodents found globally. Humans, not normally a part of the microbe's life cycle, are only accidentally and incidentally infected when fleas transmit the germs to them through a bite. About a dozen naturally occurring cases of human plague are reported annually in the United States, primarily in the Southwest. The disease it produces can take several clinical forms, one more devastating than the next.

The Black Death is more properly called *bubonic plague*—deriving its name from the greatly enlarged lymph nodes, or buboes, that are its most characteristic and recognizable feature. Although lymph glands of the neck and armpits may be involved as well, it is most commonly the inguinal nodes that present as spongy, red, and incredibly painful, swelling to the size of eggs. (*Boubon* is Greek for "groin.")

Clinical symptoms will appear two to ten days after infection, with a typical incubation period of four or five days. Malaise, headache, and high fever accompany arrival of the tender buboes, and are quickly followed by widespread hemorrhaging that darkens the skin—the Black Death has begun. In its mildest clinical form, bubonic plague will wipe out half of its victims. If the bacilli invade the bloodstream, they cause a poisoning or septicemia. This septicemic form of plague results in delirium and rapid death in 75 percent of cases.

Once the circulatory system is breached, *Y. pestis* travels easily throughout the body, infecting many organs. If there is extensive lung involvement, the pneumonic form of plague occurs. High fever, cough, and chest pain are prominent features, with the patient producing a bloody sputum. There is often gastrointestinal distress—vomiting, abdominal pain, and diarrhea—as well. Mortality is nearly 100 percent, with rapid respiratory and circulatory collapse.

In its bubonic and septicemic forms, plague is a highly lethal disease, and one of great concern to biodefense experts. It is not, however, infectious through casual person-to-person contact until and unless it turns pneumonic. Then plague becomes the nightmare of a smallpox epidemic, spreading with the ease of a whispered word.

The devastating plague pandemics of the past were most certainly of the pneumonic form. And it is this manifestation of *Y. pestis* infection that terrorists will attempt to create, through release of an aerosolized preparation, if plague is their bioweapon of choice. As an aerosol the incubation period is also shortened and disease could result within one to three days.

If terrorists are ready and willing to die for their cause, as many appear to be, they can even infect themselves and then enter an unsuspecting nation, spreading disease and death with each breath before they themselves succumb. Where there is a will, there is a way.

Pneumonic plague would initially resemble other severe respiratory illnesses, but would quickly be distinguished by the sudden development of life-threatening respiratory failure, sepsis, and shock. As in all cases of infectious diseases, early detection is critical to prevent widespread contagion. This is especially true for pneumonic plague due to the rapidity with which the disease progresses. Clinical assessment of plague made by the attending physician must be followed up by the proper diagnostic lab tests. Most important, all suspected as well as confirmed cases need to be reported immediately to state and local health departments as well as the CDC.

As with *B. anthracis*, a wide range of antibiotics can successfully treat all forms of plague. Doxycycline, tetracycline, and ciprofloxacin are all very effective if treatment begins within twenty-four hours of onset of symptoms and is continued for ten to fourteen days. For asymptomatic persons who may have been exposed to the germ, a postexposure prophylactic course of antibiotics for seven days is recommended. To date, there is an effective vaccine against the flea-borne bubonic form of plague, but it does not prevent development or spread of pneumonic plague.

Pneumonic plague, which is of most concern as a bioweapon, is spread through the release of aerosol droplets during a cough or sneeze. Thankfully, these droplets are typically greater than five microns and fall to the ground fairly quickly. A person standing more than five feet from a plague sufferer is most likely out of the effective range of infection. People in areas of contagion might also consider the wearing of simple surgical masks, since they are a sufficient barrier to the large, germ-packed droplets. Unfortunately, these masks offer little protection against the tiny spores of anthrax, or the even tinier smallpox virus—germs that require the more sophisticated filtration of a respirator called the N95.

Botulism

About two hundred years ago scattered cases of muscle weakness and respiratory failure appeared in Germany, Scandinavia, and Russia. The condition, which could quickly turn fatal, was traced to consumption of sausage and fish. It came to be called *botulism*, from the Latin word for sausage, *botulus*.

Botulism is a severe form of food poisoning caused by the incredibly powerful toxin of a spore-forming bacterium, *Clostridium botulinum*. It is a bug that can only grow in the absence of oxygen—what microbiologists call an *obligate anaerobe*. For this reason it thrives in foods that have been improperly canned, feeding, multiplying, and producing botulinum toxin in its hermetically sealed environment. Along with toxin, *C. botulinum* releases gases that swell the cans that contain it—a telltale sign of spoiled food within. It has long been the nightmare of homemakers, always on the alert for these "puffed out" cans when shopping for groceries.

Today naturally occurring botulism results in one or two dozen fatalities in the United States annually. Because illness is the consequence of ingested toxins, and no infection is established, it is not a transmissible disease. This, however, did not stop Saddam Hussein from making botulinum toxin one of his favorite weapons, stockpiling and weaponizing it by the ton. It did not stop the Japanese terrorist group Aum Shinrikyo from dispersing the toxin as an aerosol at multiple sites in downtown Tokyo three separate times—all assaults abortive.

The attraction of botulinum toxin as a bioweapon is its ease of manufacture and its lethality—a fatal dose for humans being measured in billionths of a gram. Quantities capable of killing are so infinitesimal that they are insufficient to elicit an immune response. It also appears that the toxin itself has a method of suppressing antibody production. Hence, immunity does not follow survival of such poisoning.

Botulinum toxin is a neurotoxin. All of the most potent biologically derived poisons are. The deadliest snake venoms are neurotoxins, as are the subcutaneous secretions of the South American arrow-poison frog, possibly the most powerful poison in the animal kingdom. Neurotoxins do their damage by acting on nerve endings. Botulinum's claim to fame is its ability to prevent nerves from secreting acetylcholine, a chemical that allows nerves to send impulses to other nerves as well as to the muscles they control. This results in muscles that are unable to contract—a condition called *flaccid paralysis*.

Symptoms of botulinum poisoning typically begin eighteen to seventy-two hours after ingestion. Initially there is double vision and an inability to swallow or speak properly. The muscles are beginning to lose their capacity to respond. These symptoms are followed by muscle weakness, which always descends the body, progressing from the shoulders to the upper and lower arms, then finally to the thighs and calves. Death results suddenly, when the muscles that control breathing become involved. Cardiac arrest is also a possible outcome. One horror of botulism is that the victim remains conscious and alert until the end.

A treatment for those exposed to botulinum toxin exists in the form of an antitoxin—one derived from the blood serum of a toxin-challenged horse. It is effective if injected within twenty-four hours of exposure. Unfortunately, there are seven strains of C. *botulinum*, each producing a different toxin (botulinums A through G), and each requiring its own antitoxin. Therapeutic intervention usually consists of a mixture of several of these antitoxins. The CDC maintains America's botulism antitoxin supply, and any physician diagnosing a case of botulism must contact the CDC through his or her state health department. Even with treatment, full recovery can take weeks or months, during which time the convalescing patient may require ventilator support.

A vaccine for botulism, mostly monkey-tested, has also been around for a number of years, and was even given to about eight thousand military personnel during the Gulf War. It is a preparation of the five most common toxins that have been rendered harmless, yet still evoke antibody response. Such innocuous yet immunologically active toxins are termed *toxoids*. The course of vaccination consists of three toxoid injections at zero, two, and twelve months, followed by a one-year booster. An oral vaccine, using a genetically modified toxin that survives the digestive system, is presently being researched.

Interestingly, one drawback to mass botulism vaccination—other than the obvious one of needlessly placing millions of people at a slight vaccine-related health risk—is the fact that immunization would eliminate the medical uses of botulinum toxin. Although a deadly poison, the toxin of C. *botulinum* is now being used by physicians to treat tens of thousands of people suffering from neuromuscular disorders. Involuntary muscle contraction, known as *dystonias*, can cause painful and debilitating spasms of the eyes, face, neck, or limbs. But the condition can be greatly alleviated with injections of *botox*, as the medicinal preparation is called. Headaches, back pain, and even facial wrinkling have been successfully treated with localized administration of the potent poison, although the procedure must be repeated every few months to keep wrinkles from recurring. Immunized individuals, however, could not be treated with botox.

As a bioweapon, the agent of botulism is a very real threat. Our greatest fear is an aerosolized attack, for most bioterror experts feel that, its potency notwithstanding, poisoning of a water supply with botulinum toxin is highly unlikely and very difficult to achieve. The dilution factor is so great that it would require the dumping of truckloads of toxin into the reservoir of any decent-sized municipality. Inhaled toxin, if concentrated enough, would probably present symptoms similar to the ingestion form of botulism.

Botulism poison also takes, on average, one to three days to show itself. As toxins go, this is reasonably slow-acting. Nerve gas, by contrast, produces symptoms within minutes. For many other bacterial toxins, effects appear in a matter of hours. This delay allows for therapeutic intervention, but the window of opportunity for treatment is brief. If symptoms of double vision or difficulty in swallowing or speaking occur, an immediate visit to the emergency room is critical. Dr. Philip Tierno, author of *Protect Yourself Against Bioterror* and a member of the New York City Mayor's Task Force on Bioterrorism, also recommends keeping "a supply of activated charcoal tablets in the medicine chest since they can absorb almost all poisons by chemically binding the poisons to limit further harm." As a final precaution, a properly fitting face mask can be an inexpensive yet effective barrier to toxin aerosols and might be worth keeping around the house. Welcome to the new millennium.

Bioterrorism Today

In 1984 an American cult known as Rajneeshee poisoned ten salad bars in The Dalles, Oregon, with salmonella bacteria. Their purpose was to influence the outcome of a local election. More than 750 people fell ill. No one died, but many were hospitalized. Although it was the first large-scale use of germs as weapons on U.S. soil in modern times, the government took little if any action to prevent future bioattacks.

Fifteen years later, in a 1999 survey, two-thirds of Americans polled said they anticipated a serious chemical or biological terrorist attack. Then on September 11, 2001, the unthinkable happened—the World Trade Towers in New York City were demolished and nearly three thousand innocent people murdered by suicidal Islamic extremists. The terrorist assault was an atrocity, a tragedy of such magnitude that it will divide human experience into a before and an after. About a week later, with America still reeling, an anthrax bioterror incident occurred. A few grams of highly purified and lethal anthrax spores were put into plain white envelopes and mailed to federal government buildings and news media offices. When spores escaped, more than twenty people contracted the disease, five of them dying.

Coming on the heels of the World Trade Center catastrophe, the bioterror event caused nationwide panic. The anthrax illnesses and deaths were also very instructive in a number of ways. Most significant was the realization that effective bioterror need not involve tons of pathogenic agent. Nor does it require ICBMs or warheads for deployment. A few puffs of deadly microbes are all it takes to infect large numbers of people. And if the disease is contagious, which thankfully anthrax is not, those few puffs could result in thousands of fatalities.

Through the anthrax assault of fall 2001, America also witnessed how a minor bioevent can destroy a nation's sense of well-being and security. Although only a handful of people became sick and died, hundreds of thousands of people flocked to emergency rooms, fearing that a minor sniffle, fever, or rash might be the onset of a lethal disease. Many more people demanded of their physicians and pharmacists thirty- to sixty-day supplies of the antibiotics that fight *B. anthracis*. Postal offices and congressional buildings had to be shut down as medical experts and their technical support disinfected potentially exposed areas with antimicrobial gases, foams, and radiation. The cost to America's government and health-care system ran into the hundreds of millions of dollars.

The anthrax assault also made it painfully clear that the United States was, and is, seriously unprepared for biological warfare as we enter a new millennium. If the World Trade Towers aerial attack showed Americans to be asleep at the wheel in our vigil against terrorism, then we were snoring in the backseat when bioterror subsequently struck.

For starters, few doctors were able to recognize anthrax when it appeared. This is because many of the diseases of biological terrorism rarely, if ever, occur naturally anymore. In cases of infectious diseases such as smallpox or pneumonic plague, delay in properly diagnosing the illness could be catastrophic. If we are to be alert to the dangers of bioterror, first responders in the public health arena—doctors, nurses, EMTs—must be better trained to recognize the unusual. Addressing this issue, the CDC began educating the medical establishment on how to discern and quickly contain an outbreak of likely bioterror diseases such as smallpox. In a three-day seminar, public health workers learned of the CDC's emergency smallpox plan, which calls for immediate quarantine of all confirmed cases and vaccination of everyone potentially exposed to those infected. A thirty-four-page manuscript already existed, the *Bioterror Readiness Plan: A Template for Healthcare Facilities*, which provides general recommendations to hospitals for responding to a suspected bioterror event.

As of the writing of this book—nine months after the mailing of the first anthrax letters—it is also very telling that the American government, with all its scientific and military expertise, with all its intelligence gathering, still does not have a clue as to where the bacteria came from, or who prepared the highly refined and purified powder that contained the spores. Part of the problem is a function of the ease with which germs can be acquired and grown. Technically, the culturing of bacteria is no more demanding than brewing beer. But the scientific community is divided on the question of just how easy it is to weaponize these germs. Some feel that the process of turning potentially deadly microbes into a highly lethal weapon is a daunting task, and they use anthrax as an example. After culturing the bacteria in the desired quantity, the germs must be sporulated, usually accomplished through a desiccation procedure. Then there is the problem of milling or grinding the product into fine particles, preferably the size of individual spores. Along the way, the spores must be treated chemically to neutralize the electrostatic charge they naturally acquire. This prevents them from clumping together, thus enabling the spores to remain airborne and float long distances. Aum Shinrikyo, the Japanese terror cult that poisoned the subways with sarin nerve gas in 1995, tried to cause an anthrax outbreak through release of anthrax spores on at least ten separate occasions. All attempts failed, either because the bacillus was of a nonvirulent strain, or the cult was unable to properly weaponize it. They also made three vain attempts to release botulinum toxin as an aerosol. But knowledge and expertise are continually increasing globally, and past failures provide no guarantee against a successful bioattack in the future.

Which brings us to the other school of thought. Some scientists say they can "teach a terrorist group how to make devastating germ weapons from a few handfuls of backyard dirt and some widely available lab equipment" (*Germs*, Miller et al.). *B. anthracis*, incidentally, is commonly found in soil. Recently, researchers have assembled a synthetic version of the polio virus using a recipe downloaded from the Internet and gene sequences from a mail-order supply house. Although smallpox and other lethal microbes are much more complex and difficult to assemble, their future creation in a similar way is very possible (msnbc.com, July 12, 2002).

One need not even synthesize the nightmare virus of smallpox. At least a dozen nations illegally possess the deadly microbe, including Iraq and North Korea, and it can be had for a price. (North Korea is so wacky that several years ago it appointed its dead dictator as its perpetual president.) It is not unreasonable to envision either rogue state using variola as a bioweapon or selling it to a group that would gladly deploy it against the West. Saddam Hussein might even share his bioweapons bounty with a kindred spirit such as Osama bin Laden of the al Qaeda terrorist network, if he hasn't done so already. Bin Laden considers the annihilation of America and its citizens a religious duty, one he and his fanatical followers seem willing to die for.

To make the smallpox situation even more dismal, Joshua Lederberg, Nobel laureate microbiologist and bioterror maven, says, "We have no idea what may have been retained, maliciously or inadvertently, in the labs of a hundred countries from the time that smallpox was a common disease. These would be the likely sources of supply for possible bioterrorists" (*The Secret Life of Germs*, by Tierno Jr.).

With regard to other deadly potential germ weapons—tularemia, plague, glanders, brucellosis, botulism toxin, shigella, psittacosis, cholera, salmonella, hemorrhagic *E. coli*, Q fever, dengue, Ebola, Marburg, infectious hepatitis, several forms of encephalitis, and a host of others—the U.S. Congress responded swiftly in the aftermath of September 11, 2001, enacting bills that significantly tightened security both on the deadly germs that were available for sale and distribution, and on personnel who may have access to such pathogens. Laws were promulgated that required everyone working with such microbes or their toxins to register with the federal government. Unfortunately, other countries do not have such stringent controls in place, and world safety and security is only as strong as its weakest link.

Yet another concern is the availability of vaccines and antibiotics to prevent and treat possible bioterror diseases. Before the tragic events of fall 2001, America was in dreadfully short supply of both. But things changed in a hurry, as the Bush administration allocated immediate funding for production and stockpiling of massive quantities of broad-spectrum antibiotics and the vaccines against smallpox and anthrax.

On September 11, a monstrous evil was unleashed upon the civilized world. It was a wake-up call that did not go unheeded. But answering that call would prove to be very costly. The United States' budget for national defense increased dramatically and a new Office of Homeland Security was created. Monies appropriated to counter the threat of biological terrorism more than quadrupled, skyrocketing from a paltry $1.4 billion in 2002 to nearly $6 billion the following year. In addition to replenishing our reserves of established antibiotics and vaccines, funds were allocated to the NIH, CDC, and other agencies for basic and applied research into bioterror detection, prevention, and treatment. The search proceeded, full-steam ahead, for new antiviral and antibacterial drugs, as well as vaccines against lethal infections that pharmaceuticals will not touch. Even the vaccines we presently use for bioterror threats such as anthrax and smallpox must be improved, making them safer and more effective.

Marketers say that sex sells. Well, sex has nothing on fear, and the events of September 11, 2001, were nothing short of terrifying. Not surprisingly, following the terrorist release of anthrax spores in America, federal, state, and local health-care facilities received huge influxes of capital to improve their capacities to recognize and respond in a coordinated fashion to a bioattack. A computerized network was established to keep hospitals throughout the nation, as well as the CDC, apprised of unusual symptoms and/or illnesses cropping up anywhere in the country.

Shoring up the public health infrastructure, through improved surveillance and treatment of deadly infections, will be of great benefit to all Americans regardless of whether a bioterror assault occurs, for it allows a more effective response to natural outbreaks as well. It is this "dual use" feature of a reinforced public health system that makes the additional spending a win/win situation. History has shown that we pay for what we need. We certainly need this, and the appropriations are long overdue.

The Defense Advanced Research Projects Agency (DARPA), an arm of the Pentagon, also saw its budget swell. DARPA underwrites cutting-edge scientific research, much of it addressing the concerns and fears of bioterrorism. Several futuristic projects of DARPA include the development of

- A single, multivalent vaccine that will immunize against a multitude of lethal diseases such as plague, anthrax, and tularemia

- Detergents that kill a wide spectrum of germs quickly and efficiently, to be sprayed on people potentially contaminated with pathogens
- Aerosol-based vaccines that can be sprayed over many square miles; mere inhalation could confer immunity

With regard to aerosol-based protection, Dr. Ken Alibek, the former Biopreparat chief now working in America, announced in May 2002 the creation of an inhaler that stimulates the mucous membranes' nonspecific immune response. After a bioattack, people would use the inhaler every five or six days to ratchet up short-term generalized immunity. Employing immune system chemical messengers called *cytokines*, the therapy could in theory protect a person from any pathogen. Very different from a vaccine, which works against a specific type of microbe, the "one-size-fits-all" protective spray could be ready by 2004, according to Alibek.

But until such time as a means of conferring blanket protection is realized, detecting specific airborne agents released by terrorists is critical to a rapid and effective response. Devices designed to do precisely that have been around since the Persian Gulf War, but the science of biodetection was, at that time, in its infancy. The equipment was bulky and unwieldy and not at all accurate, giving constant false positives. It is a daunting task to create an instrument capable of "sniffing out" and identifying a specific pathogen amidst all the background noise of aerosolized dust, pollen, mold spores, and other particulates in any given air sample. Even clean air has billions of harmless germs that are nearly impossible for detectors to distinguish from the deadly ones. That notwithstanding, devices are now being assembled that employ DNA fingerprinting to identify suspect microbes. In 2001, the Department of Energy's Lawrence Livermore National Lab in central California reported the construction of a two-pound, battery-operated device that could fit in a small briefcase and identify germs in seven minutes. Cepheid's detector, another DNA analyzer the size of a bread box, can allegedly signal the presence of such pathogens as anthrax, Q fever, and deadly staphylococcus germs.

The Block II Chemical and Biological Mass Spectrometer uses an entirely different technology to discern the presence of airborne pathogens. It sucks up air and then measures the mass of suspended particles to identify them. Once perfected it will be able to test for the most worrisome biological and chemical agents—anthrax, smallpox, and poisonous gases such as the nerve agent sarin. These cutting-edge detectors await proper field testing, as this book goes to print, and are one to several years away from being battle-ready.

The Massachusetts Institute of Technology and Johns Hopkins Center for Biodefense Studies are also pursuing real-time diagnostic tools that can quickly identify infected persons. MIT's project, dubbed the "canary chip" for those sacrificial coal mine birds of yesteryear, is a glass chip that contains genetically engineered white blood cells from mice. If a particular germ is present in a test sample of body fluid placed on the chip, the mouse cells produce antibodies that make the chip glow. It has already been used to detect hoof-and-mouth disease in animals and can be altered to spot human illnesses. In the near future, a patient will only have to breathe on a canary chip for an instant diagnosis.

In the meantime, what should one do between bioterror events? Horde as wide a variety of antibiotics as possible? Buy a hazmat suit, complete with boots and gas mask? Build an underground shelter equipped with HEPA (high efficiency particulate-arresting) filtration, capable of removing airborne particles as small as .3 microns? The answer is a simple no. This sort of panic and mass paranoia is precisely what terrorists want to create in a target population. The chance that anyone will ever need biohazard gear is slim to none, and it is not an item one picks up at the local department store. There are two classes of suits, termed Level A and Level B. The latter keep out low concentrations of germs and gas, while Level A suits work under much more toxic conditions. Civilians cannot get a Level A suit because it requires forty hours of training for safe use. Level B hazmat gear costs from forty-five to two hundred dollars and is also dangerous if not used properly.

Widespread personal stockpiling of antibiotics is not recommended, for it will only drain currently available supplies, increasing the difficulty of getting the medications where they are needed should a germ assault occur. Greater use of antibiotics in general will also be encouraged—a dangerous practice that produces antibiotic resistance in germs (see Chapter 3, "Magic Bullets").

One can keep a cheap, simple surgical-type mask available, which would afford protection against inhaled forms of certain diseases. The danger here is a false sense of security, since such face gear will not be a sufficient barrier against some bacteria and most viral particles.

It is the considered opinion of bioterror specialists that our most important defense against the insanity and inhumanity of germ warfare is a steadfast and constant vigil. The events of fall 2001 were a wake-up call, not only to governmental agencies, but to every single American citizen. Any unusual occurrence, any behavior that appears suspect must be reported to local police immediately. Hospitals should be notified of any uncommon ailments. This perpetual state of alert and readiness, of ceaseless and untiring surveillance is the price we are now compelled to pay for homeland security. A member of the Irish Republican Army summed up the situation very aptly, "You have to be lucky all the time—we have to be lucky just once." (*Living Terrors*, by Osterholm and Schwartz). But luck favors the prepared mind.

Conclusion

A wise man should consider that health is the greatest of human blessings, and learn how by his own thought to derive benefit from his illness.

—HIPPOCRATES

THE EARLIEST HUMAN or hominid ancestors are four to five million years old. Modern humans date back at least several hundred thousand years. A tick or two on the evolutionary clock, but a respectable span of time nonetheless. During those years humans have endured infectious disease. They have suffered through the great pestilences—smallpox, bubonic plague, tuberculosis, cholera, typhus, malaria, influenza, yellow fever, and others. At the dawn of human evolution we can only guess at the nature of the diseases that afflicted our ancestors.

One great "civilizing" event that produced many new and deadly infections for humanity about ten thousand years ago was the introduction of agriculture. Nomadic hunter-gatherers settled down with their domesticated animals—cattle, pigs, horses, sheep, goats, chickens—and received a healthy dose of their microbes. To quote Arno Karlen in *Man and Microbes*, "Agriculture brought humans so many new pathogens that it seems wondrous they survived." The most prevalent infectious disease, the common cold, made the cross-species leap from horses to humans four to five thousand years ago. Hundreds of other diseases have made a similar jump from animals to humans.

As populations steadily increased and big cities developed, communities became large enough to permanently sustain certain disease germs. Circulating among the people, these pathogens would always find new susceptibles to infect. Society had entered the age of crowd diseases and epidemics.

The human species has survived. Will it continue to do so in the face of emerging and extremely virulent pathogens? In all likelihood, yes. Logic dictates that if we have survived to this point, largely without the benefit of antibiotics, immunization, public sanitation, or an understanding of the germ theory or the nature of disease transmission, we will survive whatever future pestilence nature fashions to infect us with. Still, circumstances exist today that have not existed in the past, greatly increasing the survival threat.

First of all, there are more people in the world today than there have ever been—6.2 billion compared to 2.5 billion a mere fifty years ago. The figure increases daily. More people means a greater population density—overcrowding. Very often there is inadequate living space or food to support the number of people living in a given area. The economy of the region cannot provide adequate health care or sanitation. This is a recipe for disaster. Infectious diseases are spread most rapidly among individuals living in close quarters, with poor sanitation, whose systems have become immunocompromised by poor nutrition and who are unable to receive proper health care. These conditions are obviously most pronounced in developing nations, where vaccine-preventable diseases such as measles, mumps, and polio and controllable diseases such as cholera, malaria, and worm infections still kill millions of people each year.

Developed nations, however, are not exempt. In the United States it is surprising how poorly standard public health services are conducted. Some of the statistics are astonishing. In 1993 an adviser to the World Health Organization announced that the United States had fallen behind Albania, Mexico, and China in childhood vaccination. The United States ranks twenty-ninth in the world on infant mortality and an incredible forty-ninth in the world on child immunization for nonwhite children. Laurie Garrett sums it up in *The Coming Plague*: "We kill our children."

Fifty million people drink unfiltered water in America. Not surprisingly, waterborne microbes—such as rotavirus, the world's leading cause of diarrhea—continue to infect, sicken, and kill. Each year thousands of people die in the United States from infections by the familiar food-borne bacteria salmonella and shigella. The reason: improperly inspected and handled eggs, poultry, and beef.

Tuberculosis and AIDS remain serious threats in the United States, Canada, and Europe—and they are uniting in a frightening scenario that makes each much more deadly in combination than alone.

Jet travel has brought the human population—all six-plus billion of us—together. We live increasingly in a world community where no one is more than a half day away from anyone else. The doors of most nations are open to globe-trotters. It is a phenomenon that did not exist before the mid–twentieth century.

It creates a melting pot for pathogens and for disease transmission. The extremely virulent viruses emerging from the rain forests—Ebola, Marburg, Lassa—are not isolated to those areas. Air travel has brought Lassa and Ebola across the Atlantic from Africa to the United States. AIDS evolved in Africa in monkey primates and is now a global problem. The geographical barriers—oceans, mountains, and sheer distance—that once isolated an outbreak of disease, providing "regional quarantine," no longer do. To quote one epidemiologist, "We are all in it together."

And then there is bioterrorism. The battle to defeat the pathogens is difficult enough; add to that the human incentive to destroy other humans through disease infection, and the task becomes daunting, especially in light of the "global togetherness" that air travel has brought about, and the ease of manufacture and dissemination of lethal germs in today's high-speed, high-tech world.

To this point we have been lucky on all fronts. Mass infection through bioterrorism has not occurred. The most common yet potentially dangerous bacterial infections—strep and staph—remain susceptible to at least one antibiotic, vancomycin. The most virulent or most lethal infections—Ebola, Marburg, AIDS—are not easily transmitted. But what if common pathogens become resistant to all antibiotics? Enterococci that cause many ear infections are already demonstrating this capability, and they can easily pass their vancomycin-resistant genes to other, deadlier bacteria. What if AIDS or Ebola becomes airborne and as easily spread as the flu or the common cold? Given the conditions that exist today, it is a chilling thought.

The latter part of the twentieth century brought, along with extensive air travel, an unprecedented tampering with the environment. Governments are learning the hard way that dam building, deforestation, and the like all create new opportunities for microbes and their natural hosts to interact with humans. In the case of Lyme disease it was not the *de*forestation, but *re*forestation of treeless tracts of land in New England that brought us into intimate contact with the deer tick. Pretty, wooded suburban areas were created that attracted people as well as deer and rodents. The Lyme bacterium was not newly evolved—sporadic cases of Lyme disease had appeared for decades—but the disease became epidemic when changed environments afforded the bacterium new opportunity to infect.

In short, any sort of ecological change engenders a risk of disease to humans. Legionnaires' disease was another "new" ailment that struck as an epidemic in 1976, killing 34 of 221 people who fell ill. But the Centers for Disease Control and Prevention (CDC) investigation of frozen blood samples from unusual or unexplained pneumonias revealed that *Legionella pneumophila* had been around causing occasional and isolated cases of disease since 1947 or earlier. It was, however, the introduction of artificial environments in the form of cooling towers and hot tubs that bred and released *Legionella* into the air. It is now common throughout the world and is a significant cause of hospital pneumonia.

"To write about infectious disease is almost to write about something that has passed into history." These words were expressed by Nobel Prize–winning virologist Sir Macfarlane Burnet in 1962 (*A Dancing Matrix*, Robin Marantz Henig). Clearly he was mistaken. Forty-odd years later the message is evident: we must maintain a constant vigil. It has been estimated that improved public sanitation has extended the average life expectancy in the United States twenty years, and the advent of antibiotics and other drugs another ten. These efforts must continue and be broadened to the world stage. Programs must be implemented nationwide and worldwide by organizations such as WHO, the NIH, and the CDC to vaccinate people and to provide and properly administer antibiotics and chemotherapies. Improvements must be made in living conditions and public sanitation—especially water and food supplies. Global computer information networks must be set up to provide surveillance of infectious disease outbreaks, patterns of transmission, and mortality. Statistics must be collected and evaluated continually. And we must be more respectful of our environment and tread on it more lightly.

It is a task much easier said than done. The commitment in money and manpower would be enormous and could be accomplished only with worldwide cooperation. Richer nations would have to shoulder the greater load financially. But there is no alternative. To quote from an article in the *New York Times* (June 10, 1994), "The devastating appearance of AIDS as a worldwide epidemic put this generation on notice that it could face new or rapidly emerging threats from infectious disease. The resurgence of tuberculosis has reminded us that diseases once vanquished can return with a vengeance. These are horrible reminders that the fight against pathogens is never over."

There is little doubt that the fourth horseman—pestilence—has saddled up and is charging at us with lance poised. Hopefully we can parry his thrusts.

Bibliography and Suggested Readings

Books, Periodicals, and Newspapers

"Agency Cites Urgent Need to Fight Increase in TB." *New York Times*, 16 November 1993, sec. C, p. 8.

Altman, Lawrence K., M.D. "F.D.A. Experts Back a Vaccine Against Lyme." *New York Times*, 27 May 1998, sec. A, p. 1.

Altman, Lawrence K., M.D. "4 States Watching for Brain Disorder." *New York Times*, 9 April 1996, sec. C, p. 12.

Altman, Lawrence K., M.D. "Mad Cow Epidemic Puts Spotlight on Puzzling Human Brain Disease." *New York Times*, 2 April 1996, sec. C, p. 4.

Altman, Lawrence K., M.D. "Tuberculosis Vaccine Found Surprisingly Effective in Study." *New York Times*, 2 March 1994, sec. C, p. 14.

"Antibiotic Misuse Could Create a Public Health Nightmare." *USA Today* 123, no. 2593, p. 16.

Ariza, Luis Miguel. "Facelift." *Scientific American* 286, no. 5 (May 2002): 25.

Asimov, Isaac. *Biographical Encyclopedia of Science and Technology*, 2nd rev. ed. New York: Doubleday & Company, Inc., 1982.

Audesirk, Gerald and Teresa. *Biology: Life on Earth*, 3rd ed. New York: Macmillan Publishing Company, 1993.

"Bacteriophages Offer Alternative to Antibiotics." *Today's Science on File* 8, no. 12 (August 2000): 310–11.

Baltimore, David. "HIV Vaccines: Prospects and Challenges." *Scientific American* 279, no. 1 (July 1998): 98–103.

Barbour, Alan G. *Lyme Disease: The Cause, the Cure, the Controversy*. Baltimore: Johns Hopkins University Press, 1996.

Bartlett, John G., and Richard D. Moore. "Improving HIV Therapy." *Scientific American* 279, no. 1 (July 1998): 84–87.

Bauler, Bradley C. "River Blindness Cure in Sight." *Americas* 47, no. 4 (July/August 1995): 2–5.

Beardsley, Tim. "Better Than a Cure." *Scientific American* 272, no. 1 (January 1995): 88–95.

Beardsley, Tim. "Fighting All the Time." *Scientific American* 272, no. 4 (April 1995): 26–27.

Beardsley, Tim. "Paradise Lost?" *Scientific American* 267, no. 11 (November 1992): 18.

Begley, Sharon. "AIDS at 20." *Newsweek*, 11 June 2001, 34–41.

Begley, Sharon, et. al. "The End of Antibiotics." *Newsweek*, 28 March 1994, 46–51.

Begley, Sharon, and Adam Rogers. "Unmasking Bioterror." *Newsweek*, 8 October 2001, 20–28.

Belluck, Pam. "Severe Infection Cited in Queens Boy's Death." *New York Times*, 5 April 1995, sec. B, p. 1.

Benenson, Abraham S., ed. *Control of Communicable Diseases in Man*, 15th ed. Washington, D.C.: American Public Health Association, 1990.

Biddle, Wayne. *A Field Guide to Germs*. New York: Anchor Books, 2002.

Bleiweiss, John D., M.D. *When to Suspect Lyme Disease*. Courtesy of HoMed Lyme Care Center, April 1994.

Bradsher, Keith. "The Only U.S. Laboratory for the Anthrax Vaccine Says Production Will Be Delayed." *New York Times*, November 12, 2001, p. B7.

Bricklin, Mark. "The Promise of Nature's Pharmacy." *Prevention* 46, no. 3 (March 1994): 46–50.

Burrascano, Joseph J., Jr., M.D. *Managing Lyme Disease*, 10th ed. Courtesy of HoMed Lyme Care Center, February 1995.

Bylinsky, Gene. "The New Fight Against Killer Microbes." *Fortune*, 5 September 1994, 74–82.

Caldwell, Mark. "The Long Shot." *Discover,* August 1993.

Caldwell, Mark. "Prokaryotes at the Gates." *Discover,* August 1994: 45–50.

Caldwell, Mark. "Vigil for a Doomed Virus." *Discover* 13, no. 3 (March 1992): 50–56.

Cantwell, Michael F., M.D., M.P.H., et. al. "Epidemiology of Tuberculosis in the United States, 1985 Through 1992." *JAMA* 272, no. 7 (17 August 1994): 535–39.

Carey, John. "Cipro, Now for the Downside." *BusinessWeek*, 5 November 2001, 41.

Cartwright, Frederick F., and Michael Biddiss. *Disease and History*. New York: Sutton Pub., 2000.

Casagrande, Rocco. "Detecting Anthrax." *Scientific American* 286, no. 3 (March 2002): 55.

CDC report. "Prevalence of Penicillin-Resistant *Streptococcus pneumoniae*—Connecticut, 1992–1993." *JAMA* 271, no. 20 (25 May 1994): 1572.

Christensen, Demaris. "Another Look at the TB Vaccine: Should the United States Use BCG Widely?" *Science News* 145, no. 25 (18 June 1994): 393.

Clark, Cathy. "Four Tropical Diseases Can Be Eliminated." *Malaria and Tropical Disease Weekly*, 5 May 1997, 9.

Cohen, Jon. *Shots in the Dark: The Wayward Search for an AIDS Vaccine*. New York: W. W. Norton and Co., 2001.

"Common Bacteria Said to Be Turning Untreatable." *New York Times*, 20 February 1994, National section, p. 24.

Conner, Steve, and Sharon Kingman. *The Search for the Virus* 2nd ed. London: Penguin Books, 1989.

Cowley, Geoffrey. "Cannibals to Cow: The Path of a Deadly Disease." *Newsweek*, 12 March 2001, 52–60.

Cowley, Geoffrey. "The Endless Plague." *Newsweek*, 11 January 1993, 56–59.

Cowley, Geoffrey. "A Small Bug with a Big Appetite." *Newsweek*, 20 June 1994, 30.

Cowley, Geoffrey, et. al. "Tuberculosis: A Deadly Return." *Newsweek*, 16 March 1992, 52–57.

Dajer, Tony. "Blackwater Fever." *Discover* 13, no. 5 (May 1992): 78–80.

Daly, Michael. "Doc Battles Killer Bug." *New York Daily News*, 11 April 1995, p. 3.

Dam, Gerard Ten. "BCG—a Partial Solution." *World Health* 46, no. 4 (July/August 1993): 15.

"Debating the Destruction of a Killer." *Today's Science on File* 8, no. 3 (November 1999): 73–76.

deKruif, Paul. *Microbe Hunters*. New York: Harcourt, Brace and Company, 1933.

Desowitz, Robert. *The Malaria Capers: More Tales of Parasites and People, Research, and Reality*. New York: W. W. Norton and Co., 1993.

Desowitz, Robert. *New Guinea Tapeworms and Jewish Grandmothers*. New York: W. W. Norton and Co., 1981.

Diamond, Jared. "The Arrow of Disease." *Discover* 13, no. 10 (October 1992): 64–73.

Dixon, Bernard. *Power Unseen: How Microbes Rule the World*. Oxford: W. H. Freeman/Spektrum, 1994.

"Doctor Discovers Ebola Treatment." *Today's Science on File* 8, no. 11 (July 2000): 288.

Drexler, Madeline. *Secret Agents: The Menace of Emerging Infections*. Washington, D.C.: Joseph Henry Press, 2002.

"Drug Resistant Germ Shows Up in U.S." *New York Times*, 22 August 1997, sec. A, p. 20.

Dubos, René. *Pasteur and Modern Science*. New York: Doubleday & Company, Inc.,1960.

Elmer-DeWitt, Philip. "Reliving Polio." *Time*, 28 March 1994, 54–55.

Epstein, Paul R. "Is Global Warming Harmful to Health?" *Scientific American* 282, no. 8 (August 2000): 50–57.

Ewald, Paul W. *Plague Time: How Stealth Infections Cause Cancers, Heart Disease, and Other Deadly Ailments*. New York: The Free Press, 2000.

Ezzell, Carol. "Captain of the Men of Death." *Science News* 143, no. 6 (6 February 1993): 90–92.

Ezzell, Carol. "Hope in a Vial." *Scientific American* 286, no. 6 (June 2002): 38–45.

Fallon, Brian, M.D., et. al. *The Neuropsychiatric Manifestations of Lyme Borreliosis*. Courtesy of HoMed Lyme Care Center. N.d.

Farmer, Paul. "TB Superbugs: The Coming Plague on All Our Houses." *Natural History* 108, no. 3 (April 1999): 46–53.

Fettner, Ann Giudici. *The Science of Viruses*. New York: William Morrow and Co., 1990.

Fischetti, Mark. "Preparing for Battle." *Scientific American* 284, no. 2 (February 2001): 82–83.

Fischetti, Vincent A., Ph.D. "Bulletin from Infection Control." Distributed by Infection Control, The Valley Hospital, Banta Valley Center. N.d.

Fish, Durland, M.D., and Edward Walker, Ph.D. "What You Should Know About Lyme Disease" (pamphlet). S. C. Johnson & Son, Inc., 1995.

Fisher, Jeffrey A. *The Plague Makers*. New York: Simon & Schuster, 1994.

"For Polio, the End May Be Near." *Today's Science on File* 8, no. 7 (March 2000): 192.

Franklin, Deborah. "In Hot Pursuit of a Deadly Parasite." *The Race Against Lethal Microbes—A Report from the Howard Hughes Medical Institute*. Chevy Chase, 1996, pp. 33–45.

Friedman, Meyer, M.D., and Gerald W. Friedland, M.D. *Medicine's 10 Greatest Discoveries*. New Haven: Yale University Press, 2000.

Gadsby, Patricia. "Fear of Flu." *Discover* 20, no. 1 (January 1999): 82–87.

Gallo, Robert. *Virus Hunting: AIDS, Cancer, and the Human Retrovirus*. New York: A New Republic Book/BasicBooks, 1991.

Ganley, Elaine. "Mad cow disease darkens the French dinner table." *Staten Island Advance*, 26 November 2000, sec. A, p. 22.

Garrett, Laurie. *Betrayal of Trust: The Collapse of Global Public Health*. New York: Hyperion Books, 2000.

Garrett, Laurie. *The Coming Plague: Newly Emerging Diseases in a World Out of Balance*. New York: Farrar, Straus and Giroux, 1994.

Garrett, Laurie. "A Primer on Bacteria Worrying Residents." *New York Newsday*, 11 April 1995, sec. A, p. 3.

Garrett, Laurie. "Report: Worldwide TB Cases Up 26%." *New York Newsday*, 22 January 1995.

Gibbs, Nancy. "In Search of the Dying." *Time*, 29 May 1995, 44–47.

Gibbs, W. Wyatt. "Back to Basics." *Scientific American* 266, no. 3 (March 1993): 134–36.

Gladwin, Mark and Bill Trattler. *Clinical Microbiology Made Ridiculously Simple*. Miami: MedMaster Inc., 1995.

Glausiusz, Josie. "Ebola's Lethal Secrets." *Discover* 19, no. 7 (July 1998): 24.

Gorman, Christine. "Battling the AIDS Virus." *Time*, 12 February 1996, 62–65.

Gorman, Christine. "The Exorcist." *Time*, Fall 1996 Special Issue, 64–66.

Gorman, Christine. "A New Attack on AIDS." *Time*, 8 July 1996, 52–53.

Gorman, Christine. "The Odds Grow Longer." *Time*, 24 November 1997, 84.

Gorman, Christine. "When Did AIDS Begin?" *Time*, 16 February 1998, 64.

Grady, Denise. "Death in the Corners." *Discover* 14, no. 12 (December 1993): 82–91.

Grady, Denise. "A Move to Limit Antibiotic Use in Animal Feed." *New York Times*, 8 August 1999, sec. A, p. 1.

Grady, Denise. "New Strain of Highly Contagious Tuberculosis Is Identified." *New York Times*, 23 September 1997, sec. F, p. 3.

Greene, Warner C. "AIDS and the Immune System." *Scientific American* 268, no. 3 (September 1993): 98–106.

Guillemin, Jeanne. *Anthrax: The Investigation of a Deadly Outbreak*. Berkeley: University of California Press, 1999.

Guyton, Arthur C., M.D. *Function of the Human Body*, 3rd ed. Philadelphia: W. B. Saunders Company, 1969.

Hager, Mary, and Marc Hosenball. "Mad Cow Disease in the U.S.?" *Newsweek*, 8 April 1996, 58–59.

Hall, Stephen. "Billions of Powerful Weapons to Choose From." *Arousing the Fury of the Immune System—A Report from the Howard Hughes Medical Institute*. Chevy Chase, 1998, pp. 6–29.

Hall, Stephen. "The Return of Tuberculosis—In a New, More Menacing Form." *The Race Against Lethal Microbes—A Report from the Howard Hughes Medical Institute*. Chevy Chase, 1996, pp. 7–21.

Haynes, G. W., M.D., et. al. "The Golden Anniversary of the Silver Bullet." *JAMA* 270, no. 13 (6 October 1993): 1610–11.

"Health Agency Urges TB Medication Watch." *New York Times*, 21 March 1995, sec. C, p. 12.

"Health: Brain Disease: Mad Cow." *Today's Science on File* 10 (September 2001–August 2002): 10.

Health Logue (A publication of Bayley Seton Hospital and St. Vincent's Medical Center). "Tuberculosis—What You Need to Know *Now.*" Spring 1993, pp. 4–7.

Heemstra, Thomas S. *Anthrax: A Deadly Shot in the Dark.* Lexington, KY: Crystal Communications, 2002.

Henig, Robin Marantz. *A Dancing Matrix: How Science Confronts Emerging Viruses.* New York: Vintage Books, 1994.

Hewitt, Bill, and Ellin Stein. "A Common Germ Turns Deadly." *People*, 13 June 1994, 103–4.

Ho, David. "Alexander Fleming." *Time*, 29 March 1999, 117–19.

Jaroff, Leon. "Stop That Germ." *Time*, 23 May 1988, 56–64.

Kanigel, Robert. "A Bull's-Eye on Lyme Disease." *Arousing the Fury of the Immune System—A Report from the Howard Hughes Medical Institute.* Chevy Chase, 1998, pp. 56–71.

Karlen, Arno. *Man and Microbes: Disease and Plagues in History and Modern Times.* New York: G. P. Putnam's Sons, 1995.

Kiester, Edwin, Jr. "A Curiosity Turned into the First Silver Bullet Against Death." *Smithsonian* 21, no. 8 (November 1990): 173.

Knutson, Roger M. *Fearsome Fauna: A Field Guide to the Creatures That Live in You.* New York: W. H. Freeman and Co., 1999.

Koff, Raymond S. "Advances in Treatment of Chronic Viral Hepatitis." *JAMA* 282, no. 6 (11 August 1999): 511–12.

Kolata, Gina. "A Dangerous Form of Strep Stirs Concern in Resurgence." *New York Times*, 8 June 1994, sec. C, p. 11.

Kolata, Gina. "Defeat of a Deadly Form of Strep May Lie Within Its Own Clock." *New York Times*, 14 June 1994, sec. C, p. 3.

Kolata, Gina. "First Documented Case of TB Passed on Airliner Is Reported by the U.S." *New York Times*, 3 March 1995.

Kolata, Gina. *Flu: The Story of the Great Influenza Pandemic of 1918 and the Search for the Virus That Caused It.* New York: Farrar, Touchstone (Division of Simon & Schuster), 1999.

Kolata, Gina. "Viruses or Prions: An Old Medical Debate Still Rages." *New York Times*, 4 October 1994, sec. C, pp. 12–13.

Kuchment, Anna. "Superbug Killers." *Newsweek*, 17 December 2001, 52–53.

Langone J. "Emerging Viruses." *Discover* 11, no. 12 (December 1990), 62–68.

Larson, Erik. "The Flu Hunters." *Time*, 23 February 1998, 54–63.

LeGuenno, Bernard. "Emerging Viruses." *Scientific American* 273, no. 4 (October 1995): 56–63.

Leland, John. "The End of AIDS?" *Newsweek*, 12 December 1996, 64–70.

Lemonick, Michael D. "Can It Happen Here?" *Time*, 29 January 2001, 58–59.

Lemonick, Michael D. "Guerrilla Warfare." *Time*, Fall 1996 Special Issue, 59–62.

Lemonick, Michael D., and Madeleine Nash. "The Killers All Around." *Time*, 12 September 1994, 62–69.

Lemonick, Michael D., and Alice Park. "Streptomania Hits Home." *Time*, 20 June 1994, 54.

Lemonick, Michael D., and Alice Park. "Vaccines Stage a Comeback." *Time*, 21 January 2002, 70–75.

Lesser, T. H. J., F.R.C.S., et. al. "Ear, nose, and throat manifestations of Lyme disease." *The Journal of Laryngology and Otology* 104 (April 1990): 301–4.

Levine, Arnold J. *Viruses*. New York: Scientific American Library, 1992.

Limb, Julia. "City Orders Hosps to Report All 'Flesh-Eating' Cases." *New York Post*, 11 April 1995, p. 16.

Linden, Eugene. "Global Fever." *Time*, 8 July 1996, 56–57.

Line, Les. "Ticks and Moths, Not Just Oaks, Linked to Acorns." *New York Times*, 16 April 1996, sec. C, p. 1.

Lipsitch, Marc. "Fears Growing Over Bacteria Resistant to Antibiotics." *New York Times*, 12 September 1995, sec. C, p. 1.

Loving, Jerome. *Walt Whitman: The Song of Himself*. Berkeley: University of California Press, 1999.

The Lyme Care Center. "Lyme Disease 'At a Glance' Fact Sheet." N.p.: N.d.

Lyme Disease Foundation. "Physicians: Be Alert to These Facts!" (single sheet), 1994.

"Lyme Vaccine Approved." *Today's Science on File* 7, no. 5 (February 1999): 156.

Mackey, Robert. "Ten Diseases on the Way Out." *New York Times Magazine*, 6 May 2001, 34–35.

Mactire, Sean P. *Lyme Disease and Other Pest-Borne Illnesses*. New York: Watts Franklin, 1991.

" 'Mad-Cow' Disease Scares Brits, Puzzles Scientists." *Today's Science on File* 4, no. 9 (May 1996): 193–95.

Margulis, L., and D. Sagan. *Microcosmos: Four Billion Years of Evolution from Our Microbial Ancestors*. New York: Touchstone (Division of Simon & Schuster), 1997.

Marshall, Vincent. "Lyme and Multiple Sclerosis." Courtesy of HoMed Lyme Care Center. N.d.

Martindale, Diane. "New Worries: TB, Malaria." *Discover* 23, no. 1 (January 2002): 70.

McCormick, Joseph B., M.D., and Susan Fisher-Hoch, M.D. *Level 4 Virus Hunters of the CDC*, updated ed. New York: Barnes & Noble Books, 1999.

McNeill, William H. *Plagues and Peoples*. Garden City, NY: Anchor, 1998.

Medina, John J. *Uncovering the Mystery of AIDS*. Nashville: Oliver-Nelson Books, 1993.

"Microbes Settle in the Cities." *New York Newsday*, 25 October 1994, sec. B, pp. 32–35.

Miller, Judith. "Panel Says Smallpox Stocks May Be Useful." *New York Times*, 16 March 1999, sec. A, p. 10.

Miller, Judith, Stephen Engelberg, and William Broad. *Germs: Biological Weapons and America's Secret War*. New York: Simon & Schuster, 2001.

Minall, Gail Larkin. "Prevention is best medicine against tick bites." *Staten Island Advance*, 9 June 1997, sec. B, p. 3.

Moran, Gregory J. "Biological Terrorism: Are We Prepared?" *Emergency Medicine*, November 2001, 16–34.

Nash, Madeleine and Dick Thompson. "Attack of the Superbugs." *Time*, 31 August 1992, 62–63.

New York State Department of Health: Bureau of Communicable Disease Control. "Lyme Disease." July 1988.

Nichols, Mark with Sharon Doyle Driedger. "A Swift Killer." *Maclean's* 107, no. 50 (12 December 1994): 20–21.

Nichols, Mark. "Health: Marauding Microbes." *Maclean's* 107, no. 23 (6 June 1994): 87.

Nicholson, Joe, et. al. " 'Flesh-Eater' Eyed." *New York Daily News*, 5 April 1995, p. 5.

Nicholson, Joe. "Health chief sees no 'flesh-eater' outbreak." *New York Daily News*, 11 April 1995, p. 3.

"New Compound May Block HIV's Entry into Cells." *Today's Science on File* 8, no. 7 (March 2000): 173.

Norton, Cynthia Friend. *Microbiology*. Boston: Addison-Wesley Publishing Company, 1982.

Nowak, Martin A., and Andrew J. McMichael. "How HIV Defeats the Immune System." *Scientific American* 273, no. 2 (August 1995): 58–65.

Nowak, Rachel. "Flesh-Eating Bacteria: Not New, but Still Worrisome." *Science* 264 (17 June 1994): 1665.

Nuland, Sherwin B. *Doctors: The Biography of Medicine*. New York: Vintage Books, 1995.

Osterholm, Michael T., and John Schwartz. *Living Terrors*. New York: Delta Books, 2000.

Park, Alice. "Anthrax: A Medical Guide." *Time*, 29 October 2001, 44–45.

Park, Alice. "Fighting AIDS." *Time*, 29 March 1999, 119.

Park, Alice. "First AIDS Vaccine: Better than Nothing." *Time*, 15 June 1998, 66.

Park, Alice. "Smallpox Vaccines for Everyone." *Time*, 29 October 2001, 47.

Park, Alice. "When Did AIDS Begin?" *Time*, 14 February 2000, 66.

Park, Alice. "Who Discovered the AIDS Virus?" *Time*, 29 March 1999, 118.

Patrick, Reginald. "An Illness That Wastes the Brain." *Staten Island Advance*, December 2, 2000, sec. A, pp. 1, 16.

Paul, William E. "Infectious Diseases and the Immune System." *Scientific American* 269, no. 3 (September 1993): 90–97.

Peters, C. J., and Mark Olshaker. *Virus Hunter*. New York: Anchor Books, 1998.

Peyser, Andrea. "Manhattan Doc's Agony: He Found Cure Too Late." *New York Post*, 11 April 1995, p. 16.

Pfizer Central Research. "Lyme Disease" (pamphlet). Courtesy of HoMed Lyme Care Center, 1993.

Pike, Otis. "Mad Cows and Englishmen." *Staten Island Advance*, 11 April 1996, sec. A, p. 23.

Pines, Maya. "Can AIDS be Tamed?" *The Race Against Lethal Microbes—A Report from the Howard Hughes Medical Institute.* Chevy Chase, 1996, pp. 46–53.

"Polio Effort Paralyzed." *Today's Science on File* 9, no. 7 (March 2001): 182–83.

Preston, Richard. *The Hot Zone.* New York: Random House, 1994.

Prusiner, Stanley B. "The Prion Diseases." *Scientific American* 272, no. 1 (January 1995): 48–57.

Purvis, Andrew. "Where Does Ebola Hide?" *Time,* 4 March 1996, 59.

Radetsky, Peter. T*he Invisible Invaders: The Story of the Emerging Age of Viruses.* New York: Little, Brown & Co., 1991.

Raloff, Janet. "Livestock's Role in Antibiotic Resistance." *Science News* 154, no. 3 (18 July 1998): 39.

Ramos, Joshua Cooper. "The Real Price of Fighting AIDS." *Time,* 9 July 2001, 35.

Reiss, Spencer, and Nina Archer Biddle. "The Strep-A Scare." *Newsweek,* 20 June 1994, 32–33.

"Researchers Develop Test to Detect CJD." *Today's Science on File* 5, no. 3 (November 1996): 59.

Rhodes, Richard. *Deadly Feasts.* New York: Simon & Schuster, 1997.

Rosenthal, Elisabeth. "Doctors and Patients Are Pushed to Their Limits by Grim New TB." *New York Times,* 12 October 1992, sec. A, p. 1.

Rosenthal, Elisabeth. "Flesh-Eating Illness Confirmed as Cause of Death." *New York Times,* 11 April 1995, sec. B, p. 2.

Ross, Allen G. P., et al. "Schistosomiasis." *New England Journal of Medicine* 346, no. 3 (8 April 2002): 1212–20.

Rotello, Gabriel. "AIDS Is Still an Exceptional Disease." *New York Times,* 22 August 1997, sec. A, p. 23.

Rusting, Ricki L. "Medical Lessons." *Scientific American* 286, no. 3 (March 2002): 59.

Ryan, Frank, M.D. *The Forgotten Plague.* Boston: Little, Brown and Company, 1993.

"Same Old Strep?" *New York Times,* 10 June 1994, sec. A, p. 28.

Schardt, David, and Stephen Schmidt. "Mad About BSE." *Nutrition Action Healthletter,* July/August 1997, 4–7.

Scott, Gale. "Hospitals to Report 'Flesh-Eating' Cases." *New York Newsday,* 11 April 1995, sec. A, p. 3.

Scott, Gale. "Sudden Death: Woman's Death Linked to Strep-A." *New York Newsday*, 10 April 1995, sec. A, p. 3.

Seppa, Nathan. "A New Gap in the Antibiotic Arsenal." *Science News* 151, no. 23 (7 June 1997): 348.

Shorter, Edward, Ph.D. *The Health Century*. New York: Doubleday, 1987.

Simberkoff, Michael S., M.D. "Drug-Resistant Pneumococcal Infections in the United States." *JAMA* 271, no. 23 (15 June 1994): 1875–76.

Skow, John. "Life in the Age of Lyme." *Time*, 24 June 1991, 45–46.

Smith, Jane S. *Patenting the Sun: Polio and the Salk Vaccine*. New York: William Morrow and Co., 1990.

Smith, John Maynard. "Bacteria Break the Antibiotic Bank." *Natural History* 103, no. 6 (June 1994): 39–41.

Smith-Fiola, Deborah. "Prevent Tick Bites: Prevent Lyme Disease." *Rutgers Cooperative Extension of Ocean County*. New Jersey Agricultural Experiment Station, 1991.

Sorel, Nancy Caldwell. "Alexander Fleming and Marlene Dietrich." *The Atlantic Monthly* 269, no. 3 (March 1991): 105.

Spielman, Andrew, and Michael D'Antonio. *Mosquito: A Natural History of Our Most Persistent and Deadly Foe*. New York: Hyperion Books, 2001.

Stenor, Philip. "Deadly Virus Spreads from Horses to Man in Australia." *New York Times*, 5 December 1995, sec. A, p. 12.

Stephenson, Joan. "AIDS Researchers Explore New Drug Options." *JAMA* 283, no. 9 (1 March 2000): 1125.

"Strep Throat Can Bring Scarlet Fever." *USA Today* 122, no. 2565, p. 5.

Tarquinio, Alex J. "Ten Breakthroughs." *Reader's Digest*, February 2002, 73–78.

Taubes, Gary. "Malarial Dreams." *Discover* 19, no. 3 (March 1998): 108–16.

Taylor, Robert. *Saranac: America's Magic Mountain*. New York: Paragon House Publishers, 1988.

Thomas, Gordon, and Max Morgan-Witts. *Anatomy of an Epidemic*. New York: Doubleday, 1982.

Tierno, Philip M., Jr. *Protect Yourself Against Bioterrorism*. New York: Pocket Books, 2002.

Tierno, Philip M., Jr. *The Secret Life of Germs: Observations of a Microbe Hunter*. New York: Pocket Books, 2002.

"Tiny Bubbles Blast Holes Through Microbes." *Today's Science on File* 10, no. 4 (December 2001): 105–6.

Tolchin, Martin. "Study Says Flight Attendant Infected 23 with TB." *New York Times*, 21 October 1993, sec. A, p. 17.

Tortora, Gerard J., et. al. *Microbiology: An Introduction*, 5th ed. New York: The Benjamin/Cummings Publishing Company, Inc., 1995.

"Tougher than Ever, Tuberculosis Comes Back." *Today's Science on File* 1, no. 2 (October 1992): 38–39.

Travis, John. "Viruses That Slay Bacteria Draw New Interest." *Science News* 157, no. 23 (3 June 2000): 358.

Travis, John, Elizabeth Culotta, Rachel Nowak, and Sharon Klingman. "Reviving the Antibiotic Miracle?" *Science* 264 (April 1994): 360–65.

Treves, Frederick. "The Old Receiving Room." *The Elephant Man and Other Reminiscences*. London: Cassell, 1923.

Vanderhoof-Forschner, Karen, et. al. *Everything You Need to Know About Lyme Disease and Other Tick-Borne Disorders*. New York: John Wiley and Sons, 1997.

Villee, Claude A. *Biology*, 5th ed. Philadelphia: W. B. Saunders Company, 1967.

"Viruses Fight Antibiotic-Resistant Bacteria." *Today's Science on File* 10, no. 5 (January 2002): 130–31.

Waksman, Selman A. *My Life with the Microbes*. New York: Simon & Schuster, Inc., 1954.

Wedberg, Stanley E. *Introduction to Microbiology*. New York: Reinhold Publishing Corp., 1966.

Weintraub, Arlene, and Alex Salkever. "Killer Tests for Deadly Germs." *BusinessWeek*, 5 November 2001, p. 42.

"The Wrong Fold: Prions Key to Mad Cow Disease." *Today's Science on File* 9, no. 8 (April 2001): 185–89.

Young, John A. T., and R. John Collier. "Attacking Anthrax." *Scientific American* 286, no. 3 (March 2002): 48–59.

Zinsser, Hans. *Rats, Lice, and History*. Boston: Little, Brown and Company, 1963.

Website Postings

American Lung Association Fact Sheet: Tuberculosis and HIV. February 27, 2002. (lungusa.org/diseases/tbhivfac.html)

"Antibiotic Resistance." (mirrors.org.sg/whyfiles/038badbugs/)

"Antibiotic Resistance in Microbes." (xoma.com/sci/B1_AnRes.html)

"Antibiotics from Space." March 29, 2002. (http://science.nasa.gov/head lines/y2002/29mar_antibiotics.htm?aol37519)

"Bovine Spongiform Encephalopathy (BSE)." March 29, 2001. (fda.gov/cber/bse/bseqa.htm)

Canadian Centre for Occupational Health and Safety (CCOHS): Frequently Asked Questions. (ccohs.ca/oshanswers/diseases/legion.html)

"CDC Panel Votes for Injected, Not Oral, Polio Vaccine." June 16, 1999. (cnn.com/HEALTH/9906/16/polio.vaccine.02/)

"Childhood Vaccination Information for the American Public and Parents." November 2001. (acsh.org/press/releases/vaccination112001.html)

"Children's Immunization Schedule: The American Academy of Pediatrics' 1999 recommendations for immunizing children." April 23, 2002. (FitnMagArt.asp?Catid=237&Objid={8AAF3321-9336-11D3-8102-0090277C0A31}&curpage=2/5/02)

"Dispelling Vaccination Myths: An introduction to the contradictions between medical science and immunization policy." (unc.edu/~aphillip/www/vaccine/dvm1.htm)

"Facts About Mold." February 2001. (ci.nyc.ny.us?html/doh/html/epi/epi mold/html)

"Flesh-Eating Bacteria." 2000. (holidaylectures.org/grants/lectures/biointerac tive/web_video/bacteria.htm)

"Flesh-Eating Bacteria: Facts Behind the Bug." 1998. (dreamscape.com/morgana/amalthea.htm)

" 'Flesh-eating' bug genome decoded." April 10, 2001. (http://news.bbc.co.uk/hi/english/sci/tech/newsid_1269000/1269157.stm)

"Frequently asked questions about TB." November, 2001. (cdc.gov/nch stp/tb/faqs/qa.htm)

"General Info: General Questions about Legionnaires' Disease." June 30, 2000. (legionella.org/general_info.htm)

Grant, Amy. "Streptococcus A—Necrotizing Fasciitis." June 15, 1994. (emergency.com/strep-a.htm)

"Guinea Worm." 2001 update. (cartercenter.org/guineaworm.html)

Hernan, Patrick. "Flesh-eating bacteria kills elderly woman." *Post-Gazette News* (Pittsburgh, PA), March 18, 1998. (post-gazette.com/region state/19980318bmead5.asp)

Hernandez, Valerie. "Stachybotrys' Blame for Illnesses Debated." *Milwaukee Journal Sentinel*, July 7, 2001. (jsonline.com/homes/build/jul01/moldsid08970601.asp)

"HIV, TB and Malaria—Three Major Infectious Disease Threats." July 2000. (who.int/inf-fs/en/back001.html)

"Immunization Protects Children: 2002 Immunization Schedule." 2002. (aap.org/family/parents/immunize.htm)

"Information: Facts on Hepatitis B." October 8, 2001. (hepb.org/info.html)

"Introducing MMV—Medicines for Malaria Venture." November 1999. (who.int/inf-fs/en/factxxx.html)

Jackson, Megan C. "Group A Streptococcus." February 7, 2002. (http://justice.loyola.edu/~klc/BL472/GAS/)

Johannes, Laura, and Laurie McGinley. "Search for Better Anthrax Vaccine Increases" *Wall Street Journal*. October 19, 2001. (anthraxvaccine.org/Johannes.html)

Laino, Charlene. "New hope on HIV vaccine front." MSNBC, Barcelona, July 11, 2002. (http://msnbc.com/news/778794.asp)

Leduc, James W., and Peter B. Jahrling. "Strengthening National Preparedness for Smallpox: An Update." *Emerging Infectious Disease Journal* 7, no. 1 (January–February 2001). (cdc.gov/ncidod/eid/vol7 no1/ leduc.htm)

"Legionellosis: Legionnaires' Disease (LD) and Pontiac Fever." June 20, 2001. (cdc.gov/ncidod/dbmd/diseaseinfo/legionellosis_g.htm)

Legionnaires' Disease Fact Sheet. June 3, 2000. (multiline.com.au/~mg/legion1.html)

Legionnaires' Disease Fact Sheet. June 3, 2000. (multiline.com.au/~mg/legion2.html)

Legionnaires' Disease Fact Sheet. June 3, 2000. (multiline.com.au/~mg/legion5.html)

Legionnaires' Disease Fact Sheet. June 3, 2000. (multiline.com.au/~mg/legion6.html)

"Legionnaires' Disease: FAQ." January 25, 2002. (http://hcinfo.com/ldfaq.htm)

Livni, Ephrat. "Vaccine Victims? The Controversy Surrounding SmithK-line Beecham's LYMErix." May 17, 2000. (http://abcnews.go.com/sections/living/DailyNews/lyme_vaccine0516.html)

"Lymphatic Filariasis." 2001 update. (cartercenter.org/lymphatic.html)

MEDLINEplus Health Information Fact Sheet on Lyme disease. January 2, 2002. (http://medlineplus.nlm.nih.gov/medlineplus/ency/article/001319.htm)

MEDLINEplus Health Information Fact Sheet on Lyme disease—primary. January 2, 2002. (http://medlineplus.nlm.nih.gov/medlineplus/ency/article/000670.htm)

MEDLINEplus Health Information Fact Sheet on Lyme disease—secondary. January 2, 2002. (http://medlineplus.nlm.nih.gov/medlineplus/ency/article/000625.htm)

MEDLINEplus Health Information Fact Sheet on Lyme disease—tertiary. January 2, 2002. (http://medlineplus.nlm.nih.gov/medlineplus/ency/article/000669.htm)

MEDLINEplus Health Information Fact Sheet on Lyme Disease Vaccine (Systemic). August 15, 2001. (nlm.nih.gov/medlineplus/druginfo/lymediseasevaccinesystemic203759.html)

Nelson, Berlin D. "*Stachybotrys chartarum*: The Toxic Indoor Mold." November 2001. (apsnet.org/online/feature/stachybatrys)

"New York Recommended Childhood Vaccination Schedule." February 2002. (health.state.ny.us/nysdoh/immun/schedul.htm)

"Notice to Readers Availability of Updated HIV Treatment Guidelines." *Morbidity and Mortality Weekly Report (MMWR)*. June 4, 1999. (cdc.gov/mmwr/prebiew/mmwrhtml/mm4821a7.htm)

"Only a Fraction of TB Patients Get the Best Care." March 22, 2002. (who.int/inf/en/pr-2002-21.html)

Preston, Richard. "The Demon in the Freezer." *The New Yorker*, July 12, 1999. (http://cryptome.org/smallpox-wmd.htm)

"Riverblindness." 2001 update. (cartercenter.org/riverblindness.html)

"Schistosomiasis." 2001 update. (cartercenter.org/schisto.html)

"Scientists build polio virus in lab." Associated Press, Washington, D.C., July 11, 2002. (http://msnbc.com/news/779006.asp)

Simao, Paul. "Global Tuberculosis Epidemic Fuels US Trend." Reuters, February 8, 2002. (nlm.nih.gov/medlineplus/news/fullstory_6094.html)

"Smallpox Eradication: A Past Success—a Bridge to the Future." (cdc.gov/od/ogh/smallp05.htm)

"*Stachybotrys chartarum*: An Infosheet." April 1997. (cal-iaq.org/LAY MEM97.html)

"*Stachybotrys chartarum (atra)*—What You Need to Know." (idph.state. il.us/envhealth/factsheet/stachybotrys.htm)

"*Stachybotrys*: Factsheet." April 15, 1997. (http://hlunix.hl.state.ut.us/ els/epidemiology/envepi/eep-stac.html)

"Tuberculosis Fact Sheet." July 1999. (niaid.nih.gov/factsheets/tb.htm)

"Tuberculosis Vaccines: State of the Science." May, 2001. (niaid.nih.gov/ dmid/tuberculosis/tbvaccine.htm)

"West Nile Virus." (ci.nyc.ny.us/html/doh/html/wnv/wnv1-01.html)

"West Nile virus." National Centers for Infectious Diseases, Division of Vector-Borne Infectious Diseases. (cdc.gov/ncidod/dvbid/westnile/ index.htm)

"West Nile Virus—General Information on West Nile Virus." February 2002. (ci.nyc.ny.us/html/doh/html/wnv/wnvfaq1.html)

"West Nile Virus—Symptoms and Care." July 2001. (ci.nyc.ny.us/html/ doh/html/wnv/wnvfaq11.html)

Index

About the Authors

BARRY E. ZIMMERMAN is a graduate of Brooklyn College and has a master of science degree in microbiology from Long Island University. He has taught biology, chemistry, physics, astronomy, and medical techniques in the New York City public school system for thirty-six years and presently teaches at the West Windsor–Plainsboro District in New Jersey. He has also written curricula on science at the secondary school level for the New York City Board of Education. He resides with his family in Staten Island, New York.

David J. Zimmerman is a graduate of Brooklyn College and has a master of science degree in microbiology from Long Island University. He has taught biology, zoology, physics, and health careers in the public school system of New York City for thirty-five years and now teaches in the Englewood Public School System in New Jersey. He has written several articles on science for children's magazines, including *AHOY*. He resides with his family in Monroe, New York.

Barry and David Zimmerman have collaborated on two other books, *Why Nothing Can Travel Faster than Light* (Contemporary Books, 1993) and *Nature's Curiosity Shop* (Contemporary Books, 1995), which are collections of science essays. They also worked together on a textbook and resource manual in earth science, *Exploring Earth and Space* (Globe Book Company, 1992).

They are identical twins.